BREAKING THE POWER OF NATURAL LAW

BREAKING THE POWER OF NATURAL LAW

*Finding Freedom
in the Presence of God*

by
Jesse Duplantis

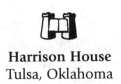

Harrison House
Tulsa, Oklahoma

Breaking the Power of Natural Law—
Finding Freedom in the Presence of God
ISBN 1-57794-224-8
Copyright © 1999 by Jesse Duplantis
P. O. Box 20149
New Orleans, Louisiana 70141

Published by Harrison House, Inc.
P. O. Box 35035
Tulsa, Oklahoma 74153

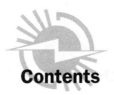

Contents

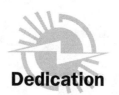

Dedication

The Lord has blessed me greatly in my life. One of the greatest blessings He gave me was my daughter, Jodi. This book is dedicated to her because without her devotion to the Lord, to this ministry and to me personally, this book would not have come into being. It is a joy to have a daughter who understands ministry the way Jodi does. From zero to twenty-seven years old, she's never seen me sick. That's why this book was written.

Thanks, Jodi, for being more than a daughter—you're a friend.

—Dad

I am the true vine, and my Father is the husbandman. Every branch in me that beareth not fruit he taketh away: and every branch that beareth fruit, he purgeth it, that it may bring forth more fruit. Now ye are clean through the word which I have spoken unto you. Abide in me, and I in you. As the branch cannot bear fruit of itself, except it abide in the vine; no more can ye, except ye abide in me. I am the vine, ye are the branches: he that abideth in me, and I in him, the same bringeth forth much fruit: for without me ye can do nothing. If a man abide not in me, he is cast forth as a branch, and is withered; and men gather them, and cast them into the fire, and they are burned. If ye abide in me, and my words abide in you, ye shall ask what ye will, and it shall be done unto you. Herein is my Father glorified, that ye bear much fruit; so shall ye be my disciples. As the Father hath loved me, so have I loved you: continue ye in my love. If ye keep my commandments, ye shall abide in my love; even as I have kept my Father's commandments, and abide in his love. These things have I spoken unto you, that my joy might remain in you, and that your joy might be full. This is my commandment, That ye love one another, as I have loved you.

—*Jesus Christ*

JOHN 15:1-12

Tap Into the Source

When I was seventeen years old, I got a job with Texaco Oil Company. The year was 1967, and the oil industry was kicking at full speed. Jobs were everywhere along the bayous of South Louisiana, and a kid like me could get a summer job working offshore on the drilling rig with no problem.

Just about every man I knew worked in the oil field. Shell, Texaco, Mobile, Chevron—all the big names—drilled out in the Gulf of Mexico, and they provided jobs for most of South Louisiana. A lot of kids my age went to work offshore, because at $2.15 an hour, it was better money than sacking groceries. And of course, you got experience in the oil industry, which would probably end up being your life's work. You got to see what it was like to live in the middle of the open sea, 150 miles off the coast on a drilling platform. You got to see what it was like to be away from home for weeks on end.

On a rig, nobody goes home at five o'clock. You're out there working six days on, six days off; seven days on, seven days off, and so forth. Sometimes it is a real adventure, especially if there is weather trouble brewing in the Gulf. For offshore workers, it isn't a big deal to see fifteen-foot swells hitting the derrick. And if a hurricane comes, well, you get right with God pretty quickly! Even atheists will cry out, "Oh, God, help us!" when they're stuck in the middle of the Gulf with 150 miles-per-hour winds whirling and rocking the rig!

For a kid, the best part about an offshore summer job was that if you saved your money, you could buy a brand-new car by the time school started. After all, in the sixties a new car went for $3,200, and you could get a beautiful, brand-new, shiny Volkswagen for just $1,795. For me, at seventeen, a new car like that was like the Holy Grail. I spent my life just hoping to get my hands on it.

That summer, I started at the bottom of the Texaco totem pole as a "flunky." They flew me out to the rig by helicopter, and we landed on the drilling platform, which was 140 miles from the coast. Now, when you're a flunky, your job is to help the cook prepare meals for the men who work on the rig.

The oil field executives know that when you keep a bunch of men out on a rig for seven days straight, you'd better keep them fed—and keep them fed well. So there was a lot of work for flunkies like me, and I kept really busy chopping, boiling and cooking. I chopped onions. I chopped tomatoes. I boiled eggs and peeled potatoes. I woke up at 4:40 A.M. to help make breakfast for the guys. Whatever the head cook said, I did. In fact, whatever anyone said to do, I did, because I was the lowest on the pole. Chain of command is law in the oil field, and if you don't follow the rules, you get shipped home. It's as simple as that.

So you can imagine my surprise when one day I went into the kitchen to peel potatoes and heard the cook say, "Jesse, the tool pusher wants to see you."

The tool pusher, I thought, *what does he want with me?*

The tool pusher was the head honcho on the rig. He was in charge of all the tools needed for drilling on the rig and was everybody's

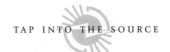

boss. He wore a big cowboy hat and blue jeans. He had a Texas accent. He smoked tobacco and looked *good* doing it. He was bad. He was the boss. And I never talked to him because, after all, I was just a flunky.

But I had done one thing especially for him that I thought he might have remembered. I peeled his tomatoes. The tool pusher didn't like skin on a tomato. He wanted the skin peeled off. So as the flunky, I got that job. I peeled those tomatoes and even got the chance to serve them to him once.

So when the cook told me the tool pusher wanted to see me, I flew out of the kitchen to see what he wanted.

Now, the tool pusher had his own little living quarters on the platform separate from the rest of us, and we called it his "shack." As I was going toward it, the radio operator stopped me. He looked me up and down, grimaced and asked, "What are you doing here?"

"I need to talk to the tool pusher!"

"What for?" he demanded.

"Look, don't get mad at me, Jack. The tool pusher wants to see me!"

I heard a voice from the shack.

"That flunky out there?"

I answered loudly and with respect, "Yes, sir!"

"Come on in here."

I walked past the radio operator toward the tool pusher's office. I tried to be discreet as I looked around. *Little red stars,* I thought to myself, *Texaco's logo. It's on everything. Hey, he's got a desk.* It was impressive.

He looked up at me and said, "Did you notice the front of this building?"

"Yes, sir."

"It's dirty. I want you to clean it."

I was nervous. I was excited. I couldn't think of much.

In a monotone voice I nervously repeated, "You want me to clean this building. How am I going to clean this building?"

"We got a fire hose over there, boy. We got a pump. Boy, we got a pump that can pump 1000 feet of casing and tubing. Just hook that pump up and wash off this building. I don't like all this junk out here. Get all this oil and dope off. I want you to clean all that up." (Just in case you don't know, *dope* is a sticky mixture of oil, gulf water and mud—it's not marijuana!)

"Can you do that, boy?"

"Yes, sir, I can!" My confidence started to perk back up.

"If you do a good job, I might make you a roustabout."

Oh, man, I thought, *a roustabout! They make $3.20 an hour. Yeah, I want to be a roustabout. I can make some money and buy myself a car!*

"Sir," I said, "when I get finished with this building, it will be so clean that you'll be able to drag your tongue across the front of it without finding a speck of dust!"

He just looked at me for a second and then said, "Well, I'll tell you one thing, we'll see about that, young man. You think you can get it done by this afternoon?"

"Yes, sir, I can!" I said and ran back to the kitchen.

"I'm not peeling potatoes today! I'm gonna wash the tool pusher's shack! He asked *me* to wash his shack!"

Now, I'm not what you'd call a mechanical man. I'm not good with tools, and I don't know how to fix much. My wife can put an engine back together with a butter knife. But me? Well, let's just say that God didn't gift me in that area.

So I was looking at the pump and the fittings and trying to find a decent hose to hook it up to. We called water hoses "hose pipes" back then. I hollered out, "Anybody know where the hose pipe is? Tool pusher wants me to clean his shack, and I'm looking for the hose! I can't find it!" A guy came over and showed me where the hoses were. He pulled one out and said, "Here, use this." I looked at the one he had selected. It was narrow and thin, and I thought, *Man, it'll take forever to clean off this building with this little hose.* So after he walked away I went searching through the stack for a bigger one.

I was digging through the tubing when my eyes landed on a big, five-inch hose. *That'll do it,* I thought as I unraveled it from the bunch. Then I looked through the fittings until I found a brass one that was just the right size. I was excited. As I cranked the big, brass fitting onto the hose, I thought to myself, *I'm going to do the best job ever!* I ran toward the pump to stretch out the hose and hook it up.

One of the roustabouts saw me going past with the hose.

"What are you doing?" he asked.

"I'm gonna wash off the building"

"With *that?*"

"Yeah."

He laughed and said, "Oh man, I've got to see this! I've got to see this!"

What's he laughing at? I thought and snapped back, "Listen here, man. Tool pusher told me to do this."

"OK. Do you want me to help you put the pump on?"

"Yeah!" I said and started stretching out the hose toward the shack.

I know now that he was thinking, *Look at this idiot.* But I was only seventeen years old. I had one hair on my chest and thought I knew something. So I grabbed my hard hat and the hose and yelled, "OK! Turn on the pump!"

Now, I didn't know it, but I was about to tap into the source. I didn't know that I was just about to break the power of natural law.

The roustabout gently pulled the valve handle down. A little stream of water started trickling out the end of my hose. But instead of continuing to turn the valve so that the water would come out fully, he stopped and looked up at me. I was standing by the shack, holding the end of the hose and looking back at him. He didn't move for second or so. Then he ran over to me and said, "If you want any more pressure, you've got to turn that valve on the pump."

He didn't want to turn the valve. So I looked at that small stream, sighed, dropped the hose and ran over to the pump. When I got to it, I looked up at him and asked, "Is it this one?" He was backing away as he nodded. I yanked down on the valve hard because, well, I didn't

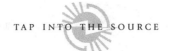

want a little stream of water. I wanted some *water*. Well, let me tell you something. I got some water—and plenty of it.

All of a sudden that pump let out a deep, whistling groan, and the hose started to shake and straighten with the force of what felt like a Red Sea of water trying to make its way through the hose.

I started to run.

Straight to the shack I went! It was a long, winding hose, and luckily I was able to grab the end of it as the water began to gush out. You wouldn't believe the water. A solid, five-inch circle came rushing out like a runaway train. The pressure was shaking me, and it was then, holding on to that fat hose, that I realized I was in big, big trouble. I could not control it.

Whack! Water hit the metal building with so much force that the whole shack shook! The hose was whipping and whirling and flapping with me on the end, and suddenly glass started flying. The water had busted out the windows, and the radio operator started hollering. I was hosing him down, and his chair was rolling back and forth in circles on the floor.

The hose was shaking my whole body, and I was sliding all over the deck as it snaked out gallons and gallons of water. I wanted to let go, but I knew that if I did, it would beat me to death. So I held on! It took all I had to keep my body on the platform.

People on the rig started hollering and running toward the pump. The roustabout who had helped me wasn't laughing anymore. He was trying to pull up on the valve to cut off the water. But something happened. He jerked hard, and between the water pressure and his pulling, the lever cracked off at the base. When that happened, I felt the force of water increase in the hose. I thought to myself, *This is it, Jack. I am going up!* And I was right.

Whoosh! I was in the air! My body jerked off the ground, and I put a death grip on the hose. That hose bumped me up and down, smacking my legs on the platform and whipping me up in the air. I was flipping and flopping and holding on for dear life. All I could do was scream.

"Hellllllllp! Helllllllp meeee! Sooommmebodddy hellllllllp!"

A grown man cannot hold a five-inch fire hose and maintain control. Now, consider what it can do to a skinny boy like I was! I didn't weigh any more than 120 pounds, and that hose had complete control of my life.

The motorman came running with a sledgehammer and started beating the pump full force, trying to turn the broken valve off. Meanwhile, I was still flying up and down with the hose and screaming, "Ahhhhhhhh!" Men were running toward me, trying to grab the hose and rescue me. They'd come close, and I'd knock them to the ground with a whirling rope of water. *Wham!* People were falling and sliding everywhere on the platform, and I was still riding that hose like a horse. Just when I thought I couldn't hold on another minute, suddenly the motorman came through! He whacked that broken valve with a sledgehammer so hard that it finally turned. Instantly, I started to fall.

Now, before the water died down, I was on top of a high-flying whip of water. I must have been fifteen or twenty feet in the air when

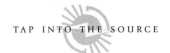
the water pressure stopped. *Wham!* I came down hard on the platform with my body still wrapped around the hose and my fingers still clenched tightly. Talk about white knuckles! The tool pusher ran out toward me and looked down at me as I lay on the platform. His brows were crinkled, and he had a confused look on his face.

Heaving with exhaustion and soaked to the bone, I looked up at the tool pusher and gasped, "It's clean, sir! It's clean!"

The tool pusher's expression didn't change. He looked up at the building. The windows were blown out, and the platform was drenched in water. He looked back at me.

"I'll tell you one thing, it sure is clean, boy. But I'll tell you this. I asked you to clean the *outside*, not the inside. You know what I'm saying?"

The radio operator came staggering out. He was aggravated and drenched to the bone.

"I never thought I'd drown at my desk," he said as he looked down at me in disgust.

"But, sir," I said to the tool pusher, "there isn't a piece of dirt on it. Just look there."

"There isn't a window in it either, boy. You almost killed that radio operator."

I was flat worn out, and I thought I was going to be fired right then and there. I didn't want to be fired lying down, so I let go of the hose and stood to my feet.

"It broke," I said, "and I didn't know what to do with it." It was all I could think of to say.

Then that tool pusher did something I had never seen him do. He started to laugh. Then he grabbed me around the head, put his arm around my neck and whispered in my ear, "I never did like that radio operator anyway. He's too smart for his britches."

"Yes, sir," I whispered back, "he is," and sighed with relief.

I Found Out What It Meant To Tap Into a Greater Power, To Tap Into the Source

That day in 1967 is one I will never forget. It was a major event in my young life and has created a memory that will be etched in my mind forever. I'm sure it's etched in the minds of a few others too!

Not long ago, I met up with a guy at a gas station with whom I used to work in the oil field. After catching up a little he asked me, "Jesse, do you remember when you blew the shed down?"

"Yeah, and I don't want to talk about it!"

He laughed and said, "People still talk about that! Some people don't believe it, Jesse. But then, they've never met you." I laughed, thinking about how one incident on a rig can eventually become legend—given enough time and retelling. I'm sure the story has changed a lot over the years out in the Gulf of Mexico, but I can tell you this—a skinny person does fly through the air if he's holding on to a fire hose! I know because it happened to me!

That day taught me a very valuable lesson, one that I later came to see as a good comparison to Christianity. I believe the story

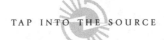

vividly illustrates a powerful truth. That day in 1967 I learned what it meant to **tap into the source.** I learned what it meant to **be controlled by a greater power.** And I found out how easy it is to be destructive when there is power in your hand. I felt what it was like to **break natural law.**

You see, there is enough power in God to fill you to overflowing and break the power of natural law. There is enough power in His Word to heal your body or deliver you from any circumstance. The power is present not only to take care of you but also to empower you to help others.

Learning How To Wield the Power of the Source

I believe that today there are a lot of Christians who are just like I was with that hose when I was kid; they've got power. They just don't know how to control their power. And in the end, they can easily fall into a state of being ineffective. Or worse, they can become destructive both to themselves and to others.

Some Christians try to get people saved, but they blow everybody out of their seats with condemnation. Others try to get people healed or show them the way out of an addictive lifestyle, but instead of harnessing their power for good, they end up knocking people down with critical words. They become ineffective. Instead of giving words of love, peace and guidance, they choose words that are laced with a slightly "holier than thou" attitude. Their words are like bright clouds, thinly lined with guilt or condemnation.

These Christians may never notice this. They think they're just "calling the kettle black," saying what is right and putting their foot down for God. But God doesn't need His children putting their foot down on His behalf unless they are doing it in love—His love.

If you've been trying to receive something from God, you may have experienced this kind of attitude from others firsthand. If so, I want you to know that God isn't into condemnation. He loves you and has enough power to heal your physical body and deliver you from any situation you may be facing today. While His kids aren't always perfect, He is perfect! He can control His power. And He wants to show you how to do it too.

You're the Valve

God has equipped us with words of wisdom, and they're all included in a book called the Holy Bible. No matter what you need from God today, it is important to know that *you* are the valve. You determine how much water comes out of the hose! And if you'll open up your heart to receive His words, I can guarantee that you will know what it means to receive a strong, steady flow of God's power in your life. You *will* tap into the Source of the supernatural—your Creator, Healer, Deliverer and Provider. You will tap into the awesome power of your Father God!

In my years as a child of God, I've come to know that nothing is impossible, because everything, and I mean *everything*, is possible with the Lord. There is *always* a way out of life's problems. And that way out *always* starts with God's Word. So that is exactly where I'd like us to look.

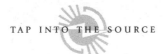
John 15 is my main text for this book, and I want you to get ready because we're about to read some Scriptures and go over some topics in this book that I believe will lay the groundwork for your understanding of how to receive from God. You don't have to be left in the dark. Right here, right now, natural law can start breaking for *you!*

Jesus Christ—The True Vine

When Jesus preached, He loved to tell stories. He knew that people could relate to real-life situations, so He used what the Bible calls parables to illustrate great spiritual truths. Sometimes with complete illustrations and sometimes with simple comparisons, Jesus used everyday situations and everyday people to get His points across.

In John 15, Jesus used the subject of a fruit-bearing vine to convey some of the great mysteries of God. From the divine chain of command to how to get your prayers answered and have joy in your life, this parable covers a whole lot. But before I dive into the fullness of it, I believe there are some foundational issues you need to know.

The Divine Chain of Command

The first verse of the parable in John 15 says, **I am the true vine, and my Father is the husbandman.**

The vine comparison really helped the people of Jesus' day understand what He was talking about. After all, they were an agricultural society. They knew something about growing grapes! Now, you may never have worked in a vineyard or picked a grape off the vine in your life, but even so, this parable was meant for *you* to hear, understand and apply. So let's think about a vine for a moment.

A vine spreads out all over. It can grow and wind around itself until it's a thick, tangled mass of branches that seems to have no end.

But as thick and winding as the plant may look, it has to start some-where. And if you'll look at a vine you'll see a thick, strong, support-ing stalk that is rooted and grounded in the earth. That is the main vine, the *true vine,* and it's what Jesus compared Himself to.

A *husbandman,* on the other hand, is a gardener or farmer. This is someone who tends the vine and takes care of all the growing branches too. Jesus compared His Father God to a husbandman.

Jesus compared people who have accepted Him as the Lord of their lives and who continue to do His will to *branches* that grow from a true vine. As Christians, we're actually the limbs of God on the earth! Isn't that a kick in the head? I've been called many things, but a limb or a branch? Only Jesus has called me that!

When the people heard Jesus say, **I am the true vine, and my Father is the husbandman,** they all knew He was using a parable to say, "Look here, people, I'm the real deal! And My Dad? He's taking care of Me and any other person who follows Me!" Now, that's my paraphrase of the parable, but I believe it is right on target. It estab-lishes the divine chain of command, the order in Christianity. This one sentence from the parable shows us that 1) Jesus is our Source and 2) God is in charge of taking care of business when it comes to His kids.

Some Vines Just Aren't True

Another foundational principle you need to know is that when Jesus said He was the true vine, He was also in fact insinuating that there are other "vines" out there that are *not* true—that are not the main vine. Jesus was saying straight up that as second in command to God, nobody was in league with Him.

As an evangelist, my job is to tell other people about the true vine. So on one hand, I feel personally responsible for letting people know that there are a lot of other vines out there. There are vines of religion, vines of theology, vines of philosophy. Throughout life there will always be people who try to make up their own rules about God. They don't want to accept that Jesus is the only way to God; they'd rather seek out their own, personal brands of "truth."

If you've ever dabbled in that kind of thinking, I must tell you this: No matter how right it sounds, if an idea doesn't base its beliefs on the whole Bible and have Jesus as the center of its teachings, it is a vine you *never* want to get tangled up in. Why? You don't want to because anything that doesn't center in on Jesus will choke the life right out of you. And I'm not talking figuratively. I'm talking literally! Hell's flames are hot. Do you get my drift?

The fact is that man's ideas have absolutely nothing to do with God's reality and His plan for man. God is in control. He won't change His truth to fit man's ideas. Man's ideas change from day to day, year to year, decade to decade and century to century. But God? Well, He *never* changes. He knew the world was round when, centuries ago, men were scared of sailing for fear they'd fall off the side of the world. Today we've got theories floating around that are just about as ridiculous as the assumption that we live on a flat planet.

But God knows what's true. He isn't theorizing. He isn't swaying the truth on account of man's flip-flopping theories. Let's face it, it really doesn't matter what anybody thinks God *ought* to be like. It doesn't matter what we think He *ought* to do or say. God is who *He* is. He said what *He* said. He made a plan for our salvation, deliverance, abundance and healing through Jesus' life, death and resurrection. It isn't up for negotiation.

Never Let an Element of Truth Distract You From *the* Truth

I don't knock other religions about their ability to help people out sometimes. I've read some of their books. After all, I wanted to know what they had to say. And do you know what I found out? Many aren't that bad. Some offer wisdom and insight about mankind. Some teach moral principles that are not unlike Christianity's. Some stress peace; others stress love. Some offer techniques to calm you down if you're having a rough day and help you get through difficult mental situations.

The problem with the books and teachings of other religions is that, as good as they sound, they *won't* get you to heaven. You see, God won't allow anyone to discount His plan—Jesus—in favor of another and still get to heaven after death—not you, not me, not anybody! God bound Himself to His Word when He sent Jesus, so He won't put His stamp of approval on a book that deceives people into thinking that Jesus' blood doesn't count.

That is why some religious books, no matter how old and seemingly important, are just like other self-help books on the shelf at the bookstore. They have elements of truth, but they aren't *the* truth. I don't care if their principles date back *before* the time of Christ—that still doesn't make them the truth! And that's the *big* difference when it comes to getting in line with God.

After all, what is the point of adhering to a religion's code if you end up going to hell when you die anyway? If I'm going to hell, I don't want to do it sticking to some nice-sounding religion's rules! Do you? No way, that's crazy!

All Roads Do Not Lead to God

No matter what represents itself as truth, the only real truth is Jesus. Jesus said, **I am the way, the truth, and the life: no man cometh unto the Father, but by me** (John 14:6). This means that Jesus is the *only* way and the *only* truth. The *only* method of obtaining eternal life with God is by accepting Jesus as Savior and Lord.

Some people refuse to accept that Jesus is the only way to God. They may say, "All roads lead to God." That sounds good to man, but God is pretty matter-of-fact about what He accepts. He didn't sacrifice His Son for nothing. What's true is true. And whether any of us choose to believe the truth or not doesn't change it.

People can make up whatever helps them sleep at night. They can pray to a tin can and make elaborate rituals of sacrifice to it for centuries, but in the end Philippians 2:9-11 assures us that *every* knee is going to bow and give honor to the true vine, Jesus Christ:

Wherefore God also hath highly exalted him, and given him a name which is above every name: that at the name of Jesus every knee should bow, of things in

heaven, and things in earth, and things under the earth; and that every tongue should confess that Jesus Christ is Lord, to the glory of God the Father.

During this life or the afterlife, it's just a matter of time before everybody's knees hit the dirt. Yours, mine, *everybody's!*

So what happens if you try to create your own way around Jesus and His teachings? You lose, both in this life and the afterlife. First life becomes confusing and empty. You wonder why you have this "void," and you seek things in life to fill it. I've seen people try to fill that void with all sorts of things. Some shift from relationship to relationship, trying to fill their emptiness with emotional highs. Others try to fill the void by striving for success and accomplishment. Still others may try to fill the void with alcohol, drugs or even food and entertainment.

All that makes for a confusing and often miserable life. But the worst part is that after a life with no *real* purpose, people miss eternal life too. Now, that's a raw deal! But God doesn't negotiate: Jesus is everyone's ticket to a life of fulfillment on earth and an eternity in heaven.

Hell Is Hot—Try To Avoid It

Some people don't believe in hell, but that's probably because they either haven't read much of the Bible, or they've read it and simply chosen *not* to believe it. But Jesus talked about hell quite a bit. He didn't want anyone to go there. You can find remarks about hell throughout the Bible.

Just how many times is hell mentioned in the Bible? At least forty times!

Here are a few that you can check out for yourself: Matthew 3:12; 5:22; 5:29-30; 7:13-14; 8:11-12; 10:28; 11:23; 13:30,38-42,49-50; 16:18; 18:9,34-35; 22:13; 23:15,33; 25:28-30,41,46; Mark 9:43-48; Luke 10:15; 12:5; 16:23-26; Acts 1:25; 2:27-31; 1 Thessalonians 1:10; James 3:6; 2 Peter 2:4; Jude 1:6-23; Revelation 1:18; 2:11; 6:8; 9:1-2; 11:7; 14:10-11; 19:20; 20:10,13-15; 21:8. Those are just some of the times hell is talked about in the New Testament.

Hell was never supposed to be for humans. It was created for the devil and his demons. But since the fall of man, those who choose to side against God in turn choose to share their eternal home with Satan. His home isn't nice. It's hot. It's miserable. And I don't care what anybody tells you—it's never, ever going to freeze over.

The best choice is to avoid it altogether by choosing to follow God's plan.

Salvation Is Easy

The good news is that making heaven your home is very, very easy. God didn't make it hard. All we have to do is accept His Son, Jesus, as our personal Lord and Savior, and *wham!* when we die, we immediately are ushered into God's home!

Romans 10:9-10 NKJV shows us how to make the transition and "get saved." Saved from what? Saved from confusion in life and from hell after death. The Bible gives us the instructions right here:

If you confess with your mouth the Lord Jesus and believe
in your heart that God has raised Him from the dead, you will
be saved. For with the heart one believes to righteousness, and
with the mouth confession is made to salvation.

This Scripture shows you how to start a new life with Jesus. I did
it in 1974, and it completely changed my life.

How God Changed My Life

As you might have heard me say in some of my sermons, I was
a rock musician in the late sixties and early seventies with a serious
addiction to alcohol and drugs. I drank a bottle of whiskey every
day—not for fun but just to start my day out. I'd do so many drugs
that I'd break out in purple splotches all over my chest. I took many
trips without leaving my hotel room.

One night I was flipping through the channels on TV before a gig,
and I landed on a Billy Graham crusade. It was being televised in a
stadium. My wife, Cathy, who had been saved a year and a half earlier,
wanted to watch it.

"I don't want to watch that garbage!" I said when she told me to
leave it on. She didn't miss a beat. She said, "Why not? He pulls in
more people than you do." Ouch. It was true, and I knew it. I didn't
care, so I left it on just to kill some time before leaving for my show.

I won't go through all the emotions I felt that night, but I will say
this—God touched my heart through that program. As an angry alcoholic and drug addict I was hanging on to some pretty heavy baggage.
And by the time Billy Graham gave an altar call, I couldn't hold on to

the bags anymore. God was working on me. Of course, I didn't want my wife to see my being affected by the program, so I did the only macho thing I could think of. I went to the bathroom. And it was there, in a hotel bathroom in Boston, Massachusetts, that I gave my life over to God. You could say that I met Jesus right at the throne!

I don't remember my exact words, but I know I said something like, "If there is a God, come into my life and change me." I wasn't playing around; I was sincere. My voice might have been a whisper, but my heart was crying out for something real.

Suddenly something broke in my heart, and I began to cry—which I never, ever, and I mean *ever*, did. I was a "man." I'd been taught all my life that men just don't cry. Crying was for wimps and sissies. But when Jesus came in and touched my heart that night, I couldn't stop myself from crying out. The tears just started to fall down my face.

Do you know what happened to me? *Jesus* came into my heart that night. The One who created the universe came down and changed *me!* He touched my heart, and suddenly something changed in me. I went from being a drug-filled angry sinner to a clean, joyful, righteous man in one night—actually, in a couple of minutes! I didn't know it right then, but He supernaturally delivered me from drug and alcohol addiction that night. I never went on another drug trip. I never got drunk as a skunk again. And that was a big deal because I'd been boozing it up for years. I put vodka in my cereal. Vodka and corn flakes—it was a good combo for me. But suddenly, I didn't want it.

Accepting Salvation—
From Heart-Change to Life-Change

Jesus changed my heart, and because of the heart-change, I started to make some changes in my life. Accepting Jesus completely transformed my life, and I know He can do the same for you. Before you can receive anything from God—whether it's healing or anything else—you've got to make that heart-change.

If you haven't accepted Jesus into your life, I've printed a prayer at the back of this book especially for you. It'll help you get going when you approach God in prayer, but you can say it in your own words. Just remember this: It's sincerity that counts. God will meet you right where you are. Please turn there now, and give your heart to the Lord.

The Bible—Your Welfare Book

If you die right after you get saved, salvation is all you really need to make heaven your eternal home. But if you have to live any amount of time at all on this planet, you will want to go beyond the salvation prayer and start using the rest of the Bible as your manual for living. I like to call it a "well fare" book—it is there for your welfare. And if you obey it, you'll fare well!

Salvation is the foundation for Christianity and undeniably the most important subject in the Bible. Although it may sound like a cliché, according to Romans 10:9-10, you really *do* have to believe before you can receive salvation.

Now, most Christians understand that without faith in God's plan, Jesus Christ, salvation is impossible. They realize that faith is a must when it comes to salvation. But sometimes they can get stuck when it is applied to other things in the Bible—like healing. When it comes to healing, suddenly everything gets complicated and wishy-washy, and in the end, a lot of people don't really know what they believe.

I can understand that. There is a lot of confusing stuff out there about healing. But the bottom line is that God really didn't make healing complex. We might, but He didn't! He lumped it in there with everything else Jesus died to redeem us from, all of which come by a substance that a lot of Christians today have really misunderstood—faith.

The Truth About Faith

Faith. Now there's a word that many actually consider to be a message that is at odds with God. But really, it's just about believing what God said.

Faith isn't a "message" really. It's not a "movement" either. While there are some ministers who seem to specialize in preaching faith, they didn't make it up. Faith isn't some new teaching. God put the "believing and receiving" system into effect, and Jesus made the term popular. Anyone can read the Gospels and see that.

The theme of faith, or trusting God, is intertwined throughout the whole Bible, from Genesis to Revelation. But even though faith appears throughout the Bible, it isn't the *only* thing in the Bible. Think about it. How many times do you read about grace in the Word? What about mercy? Or how about God's love?

On the other hand, even though faith isn't the *only* topic in the Bible, it seems to be mixed up with just about everything else in there. In fact, for faith to work at all you need to be walking in God's love. (Galatians 5:6.)

So even though faith isn't the only area you need to study in the Word, it is crucial to your success as a believer. It is important that you know about it, not just as some part of the Charismatic lingo but as a real and viable power tool for *your* life. Faith is God's key to breaking the power of natural law.

You've Got a Built-in *Substance* Designed To Connect With God's Word

Now I want you to think about it. What is it that makes you believe God's Word is true? *Faith* in God's Word. What makes you think you get righteousness by believing in your heart that Jesus rose from the dead? Faith in God's Word. What makes you think you can get salvation by confessing with your mouth Jesus as your Lord? Again, it is faith in God's Holy Word.

Why do you believe? Because something inside the very core of your being connects to the Word. You read it or someone tells you about it, and something clicks within you. You know that it is true. How do you know?

You know because God placed a substance inside you that was designed to be stimulated when confronted with His Word. What is that something? It is the amazing substance the Bible calls faith. Faith isn't floating around in the atmosphere somewhere; it's in you. The Bible says that *every* person is given the measure of faith. (Romans 12:3.)

God didn't leave you out when He was handing out faith. That is why you can read a Scripture, and suddenly it hits home. You get a "revelation," as they say. You recognize a Scripture for what it *really* means. That is when your measure of faith jumps up inside of you and says, *I see what God meant, and I know that this stuff is true!* That is when, all of a sudden, you accept it as *more* than just a fact. You accept it as the truth. You believe it. And suddenly you receive it.

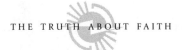

Suddenly!

For years I've said that *suddenly* is one of my favorite words in the Bible. I like excitement, and suddenly is sure more exciting than eventually, don't you think?

Regardless of how it appears, healing, for example, really does come suddenly. Again, consider salvation. Salvation doesn't take two years. It happens suddenly. The Bible says that there are some who are saved **as by fire** (1 Corinthians 3:15). In other words, they are about to bust hell wide open, but at the last minute they open their hearts to receive salvation, and *wham! Suddenly* the blood of Jesus gushes in and redeems them! *Suddenly* they are stolen from the hand of the enemy and reborn as children of God!

At the very last moment, they call on the name of Jesus, sidestep the heat of hell and are ushered into the kingdom of heaven! *Whew!* That's what you call a close call! Thank God that His blood can redeem even until the last millisecond of a person's life.

Healing isn't much different when it comes to making that connection with God.

The Word Stimulates Faith, And Faith Activates Power!

There is a *connection* that takes place when the Word of God stimulates the measure of faith inside of you. The Word of God is alive. It is living and active. (Hebrews 4:12.) And the faith you have inside of you was given to you by the living God who inspired the Scriptures we have today.

When you connect the measure of faith with God's Word, something extraordinary happens. Faith and the Word collide, and *wham!* an atmosphere for the supernatural is instantly formed. Suddenly, the power to break natural law is present.

Suddenly, you experience that mysterious thing called receiving; the time when the blood of Jesus begins to gush in, the time when the very power of God is drawn into your physical body, obliterating sickness and disease. It is a combination of faith and the Word that activates God's power within your life. And it doesn't take years to happen. It can take place in an instant.

This is why Jesus said you could move mountains with your faith. He said that if you'd only believe you could say, "Move!" to a mountain and it would fall into the sea. (Mark 11:23.) I don't believe that was just a poetic way of saying, "Major stuff happens when you use faith." I believe that Jesus used those particular words because they symbolized *your* ability to break natural law. After all, who can deny that natural law would have to be broken in order to send a mountain flying into the sea?

There Is a Huge Difference Between Mountains and Mustard Seeds

Jesus said you could move something as large as a mountain with something as small as a mustard seed. (Matthew 17:20.) Now, He used the analogy of a mustard seed because it was the smallest of the seeds people planted in His day. It is tiny. You practically have to squint to see a mustard seed. But a mountain? How can you *not*

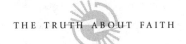
see it? You can't even see around a mountain. It's so big that you can only see one side. If it's sticking out of the sea, it is even bigger because the thing goes down into the ocean! It's so big—it sits on the floor of the ocean!

Compare that mountain to a seed so small you've got to squint to see the details of it. Big difference, right?

Well, that's the ratio Jesus laid out between faith and your problems. Even if you've got to squint to get a look at your faith, it's enough to plow through a gigantic problem you can't see around. No matter how huge, deep-rooted and twisted that problem is, all you need is an itty-bitty speck of faith to start it on its descent into the sea.

It's *Now Faith Is*—Not *Is Faith Now?*

What is faith anyway? The Bible calls faith the substance of what you hope for and the evidence of what you don't see. (Hebrews 11:1.) In other words, you're saying, "Jesus, I believe You can and will do this thing that I hope for. And because I believe that You can and will, I take Your Word as evidence that it is already done."

That's what you call trust! You're trusting that God's Word will work for you. You are trusting in it so much that you don't even consider that what you hope for *might not* happen. "Of course it is going to happen!" you might say. "We're talking about God here!" Now, if you're thinking like that, you're going in the right direction.

The King James Version's definition of faith goes like this:

Now faith is the substance of things hoped for, the evidence of things not seen. For by it the elders obtained

a good report. Through faith we understand that the worlds were framed by the word of God, so that things which are seen were not made of things which do appear.

HEBREWS 11:1-3

God used faith to create the worlds. He used it to create you! The fact that you're here at all is evidence that God had faith! That ought to tell you something!

I think a lot of people negotiate with the things of God, choosing one instead of the other when the potential is there to receive *all* from God. What happens if you negotiate around the truth that Jesus delivers? You could get stuck fighting off miserable things like depression or addiction.

And what happens if you negotiate around the truth that Jesus blesses abundantly? You could miss out on God's plan for your earthly success. You could stay broken by poverty or limit God's ability to bless others through you.

And healing? What if you negotiate around the truth that Jesus heals? Yeah, you got it. You could remain bound by sickness and the freedom of living healthy. But faith is faith, no matter whether it is put in God's power to save, deliver, prosper or heal, or if it is put in Satan's powers to steal, kill and destroy.

Some people make faith hard. Instead of trusting in *Now faith is* they say, "Is faith *now?*" They change the words and confuse themselves. But it is in black and white right there in the Bible, so don't let those people confuse you! If you hear someone say, "That faith stuff isn't for today," remind yourself of Hebrews 11:1, and then ask

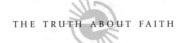

yourself, "When is *now?* Is now tomorrow? Is now yesterday?" Then answer yourself, "No! Now isn't in the past! It's in the immediate present. Now means now! It happens *suddenly. Now faith is!*

When You're Hungry, When Do *You* Want To Eat?

When you're sleepy, when do you want to sleep? Later? When you hear your stomach growling, you don't say, "Hmm. I'm starving. I think I'll eat in a couple of days."

I don't know about you, but if I'm sleepy, I want to take a nap! And if my stomach is stabbing me and growling like an animal, it can mean only one thing: It's time to chow down! Give me something to eat before I devour the next thing that moves.

You can attack sickness in much the same way. You can say to yourself, "I'm not waiting forever for my healing! I'm going to do everything in my power to get this thing done! I'm going to do my part, and God is going to do His; and between the both of us, I'm getting healed!"

It may sound kind of childlike to be demanding like that, but really, that's what it takes! If you look throughout the Scriptures you can find stories of people who were demanding and received. Jesus responds to people who have enough faith to draw from His power.

Childlike but Not Childish

Kids have a great understanding of the word *now.* That is why you hear so much about childlike faith. Think of the way a child acts, and you've got a good idea about the essence of faith. For example, when a kid sees a piece of candy at the checkout counter in a grocery store, he zeros in on it and commands you to do what? Produce!

That child locks his little mind on that candy, and buddy, you'd better *know* that he isn't asking for it next week! When is the time for candy? *Now* is the time for candy! Baby wants it now! Do you understand what I mean? If you've ever dealt with a kid having a candy fit at the checkout counter, I'm sure that you understand what I mean.

Breaking the power of natural law through faith is much the same way—it has all the elements of childlike faith and tenacity without the childish tendency toward whining and complaining. It is about realizing that power flows *now* and *suddenly* and that you don't give up if something doesn't go perfectly along the way.

Childlike faith is about sticking to it until you make the connection with God's Word and draw on the blood of Jesus. It's not about *when* you get healed; it's about realizing that by His stripes you *were* healed. (Isaiah 53:5.) You've got to know in your heart that "were healed" can change "are sick." Stop and think about that for a moment.

The grown-up in you talks away the issue. The grown-up looks at the facts so much that he misses the truth. As adults we are taught *not* to be childlike but to give up on our dreams, be logistical and never take what people say literally. Basically, we're taught to give up our childlike faith in favor of cold, hard facts and cynicism. But Jesus didn't tell us to do that. He didn't instruct us to act that way at all.

Jesus told us and showed us through His example that we should strive to have childlike faith. He showed us through His example that we should hit the root of problems instead of wading around in

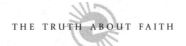
logistics. Throughout His life, Jesus continually shoved rules and regulations out of the way and spoke on the heart of matters.

If you think about it, that's exactly what children do. They don't have to know the methods of making candy in order to enjoy it! They don't care how much corn syrup it takes to create a cherry-flavored lollipop. They just grab that sucker and start licking and chewing until that thing is gone!

That is what you do with the Word of God too. You just keep taking it in until it's *within* you, until it's a part of you. You may be a person whose childlike faith is easily tapped. You may be a person who can put aside logistics and believe pretty quickly. Consequently, you may also receive quickly.

Or you may be like a lot of others who need to hear a bit more of the Word to help stimulate their childlike faith. You may need to wade through some of the "adult" thinking and get into the habit of using the childlike faith God put in you!

After all, you don't have to know exactly how an engine runs to drive a car and get where you're going. You don't have to know all about gravity and the law of lift to ride in a jet. All you really need to know is that God's Word is for *you* and if you believe it, it can simply work a miracle for you—regardless of the complications of the situation.

You Need the Prayer of Others

If you're sick, you don't have to face it alone. Not only is Jesus inside of you, but you've got people all around you who are willing to pray the prayer of faith for you. James 5:14-16 instructs you on exactly what to do if you get sick:

> Is any sick among you? let him call for the elders of the church; and let them pray over him, anointing him with oil in the name of the Lord: and the prayer of faith shall save the sick, and the Lord shall raise him up; and if he have committed sins, they shall be forgiven him. Confess your faults one to another, and pray one for another, that ye may be healed. The effectual fervent prayer of a righteous man availeth much.

In other words, the prayers of the righteous work!

There are people walking in the gifts of the Spirit in the church today—as described in 1 Corinthians 12:8-11,28—and also many good churches with pastors and teachers who believe in healing and are willing to lay hands on you and pray the prayer of faith.

Don't Be Bashful! Get Yourself to the Altar for Prayer!

I know of some people who have talked about healing so much that they're embarrassed when sickness tries to attach itself to their bodies. I know some preachers who leave their hometown when they're sick because they're afraid their congregation will find out. They're scared of what the "faith crowd" will think about them if they admit to being sick.

That's crazy. Don't let pride keep you from having other believers pray with you. You know, I believe in healing. And I'm healthy. But I've had sickness try to attach itself to me, and do you know what I've done about it? I've fought it with my faith and my will. I've spoken

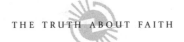
good things over myself. But I'm not afraid to say, "Hey! Pray for me! The devil's attacking my body."

Yeah, I'm a faith preacher. And yeah, sometimes I need prayer. Big deal. Nobody on this earth is perfect. Sometimes the devil tries to knock us in the head. But that isn't any reason to skip town and pretend like nothing bad ever happens. This is a way that people are robbed of one of the most important facets of healing—the power of united prayer.

Not too long ago, I had a problem in my body that was really getting on my nerves. It happened after I ate some ten-year-old Vienna sausages. Yeah, I know I should have looked at the date on the can. But my wife wasn't home and I was looking for something to munch on. You know, my wife doesn't cook much, so you can bet she hadn't been cleaning out the pantry. I found that little can of poison lurking in the back corner of the pantry.

I peeled open the can, grabbed a sausage, slugged the jellied fat off of it and went to chomping. Big mistake. That sausage tried to murder me! I got choked up and couldn't breathe. I got dizzy, the room started spinning, and I could hardly walk straight. After the initial symptoms, I still had to fight the devil tooth and nail over what that sausage did to my body! I know that eating ten-year-old sausage was my own fault, but thank God, God had grace—and here I am today!

Now, I'm not a man to show much weakness. I guess that is a product of my upbringing. I'm not one to blab my problems to people. I figure Jesus can take care of it. But sometimes you need other people to pray with you. And when those times come, I'm not above asking for prayer. Faith preacher or not, if I'm sick, I want somebody to believe with me. I want somebody to pray for me because the prayer of a righteous man avails much.

I know quite a few righteous men. But I've got one friend with whom I feel the most comfortable talking about what I need from God. He is a great man of faith whom I admire. He's older than I am and has been saved longer than I have. And he has shown me time and time again that he actually gives a flip about what happens to me. I think God must tell him when to call me and let me know he's praying for me, because sometimes I'm blockheaded and won't tell other people I need prayer. But this guy is in touch with God!

After the sausage incident, a nagging problem kept trying to surface. I'd get dizzy for no reason. I told my wife about it and mentioned it a few times in passing. Then one day I got a call from my friend. I was scheduled for a routine physical, and I was trying to avoid it because, well, I wasn't looking forward to some of the tests they do. He called me one day to talk to me about it.

This friend of mine said, "Jesse, you need to get down there to get that physical. And listen, don't worry if they find something. You've got faith. Together we can whip this thing."

I thought, *Look at this here! Somebody is calling to encourage me!*

I said, "I know, and I'm not worried about it! I'm going!"

I went and got a clean bill of health. The doctor told me I was so healthy that I was in the top 20 percent of the nation! I thought, *I could*

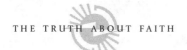
have told you that. He told me that the dizziness was an allergy and let me know that sometimes people start getting allergies in middle age.

Middle-age allergies? I thought, *Not me, Jack! I'm fighting this thing!*

So I started walking out my healing like the lepers did in Luke 17:14: **And it came to pass, that as they went, they were cleansed.** And I did it by faith, knowing that in the process I would be healed of allergies!

That is God's plan for you and me. You might be a brand-new baby Christian. You may be a faith preacher like me. You may be a person of great faith who is having a hard time receiving healing for yourself. Regardless of your position in Christ, I want to let you know that *you* can walk out your healing like the lepers and be healed in the process! *You* can walk by faith!

So don't be bashful to ask for prayer. Don't be embarrassed if something has gotten ahold of your body. So what! Be tenacious! Be bold! Have faith, and get to the altar for prayer. Let somebody lay hands on you and pray the prayer of faith. Call friends who won't poor-mouth your situation, and ask them to stand with you. God has many warriors who can stand with you in prayer.

I'll tell you what my friend told me:

"Don't worry. You've got faith. Together we can whip this thing!"

You and God can whip this thing for good!

Healing—It's for Today!

Surely he hath borne our griefs, and carried our sorrows:
yet we did esteem him stricken, smitten of God, and afflicted.
But he was wounded for our transgressions, he was bruised
for our iniquities: the chastisement of our peace was upon
him; and with his stripes we are healed.

ISAIAH 53:4,5

Did you know that Isaiah spoke these famous prophetic words
eight centuries before the crucifixion actually took place? In
this amazing passage of Scripture, Isaiah writes about the details and
purpose of the crucifixion of Jesus Christ. But as great as redemption
was, Jesus did a lot more at the Cross than take our sins away.

This passage says that Jesus suffered to bear our griefs and sorrows
too. It says that He suffered for our peace and healing as well. So not
only did He make a way for us to escape the judgement of God concerning heaven and hell, but He also made a way for us to be healed!

Jesus fulfilled Isaiah's prophecy of divine healing when He came
to the earth and went to the Cross. Matthew 8:16-17 says,

When the even was come, they brought unto him many
that were possessed with devils: and he cast out the spirits
with his word, and healed all that were sick: that it might be
fulfilled which was spoken by Esaias the prophet, saying,
Himself took our infirmities, and bare our sicknesses.

If you are at all confused about whether healing is for today, Isaiah 53:4-5 and Matthew 8:16-17 settle the issue. You don't have to wonder what the blood of Jesus did. He spelled it out right there, 800 years before it ever happened! Just as Jesus became the mediator between God and man concerning salvation, He also became the mediator between God and man concerning healing.

Jesus—The Same Yesterday, Today and Forever

In Jesus' time, religious people were always challenging Him. Today, religious people still challenge His work on the earth. Even those who agree that He is the Son of God challenge Him!

In John 8, Jesus dealt with this firsthand. He was talking to the religious people around Him about His position with the Father. He was letting them know who He was and what would happen if they believed Him. But instead of receiving Jesus' words, the people got hostile and began to challenge Him.

They even went so far as to ask Jesus if He was demon possessed. (v. 48.) With that, Jesus let them have it. He didn't hold back either. He let the truth go free! Read the chapter, and you'll get the feel of it.

One of the best parts of that passage is in John 8:56, when Jesus said to them, **Your father Abraham rejoiced to see my day: and he saw it, and was glad.**

They must have thought, *Just who does this Jesus think He is!* It really bothered them. Angrily they mocked Him and said, **Thou art not yet fifty years old, and hast thou seen Abraham?** (v. 57).

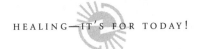
Jesus said, **Verily, verily, I say unto you,** *Before Abraham was, I* AM (v. 58).

Whoa! You would have thought Jesus cussed at them! The people freaked out and tried to stone Him! Abraham was like a god to them. And here was Jesus saying, "Look, before God even thought about Abraham, I was here!"

If Healing Is Not for Today, Then Nothing Else in the Bible Is for Today

Now, I realize that some Christians debate Jesus' present healing ministry in the earth. They say, "Is it for today?" I believe that John 8:58 proves that Jesus and His work on the earth *is* for today because Jesus Himself isn't limited to a certain space of time.

I guess you can tell that I disagree with those theologians who would try to condemn preaching on healing by saying things like, "Well, you know, miracles are not for today. And what you're teaching is all past." Some say that healing was only done then for the purpose of proving Jesus' divinity. That's what I call thorny, theological wilderness weeds! People choke out the power when they try to explain it away. But Jesus' Word is forever.

When He said, **I** AM, He proved that He *and* His work are timeless. There is no cap, so to speak, on Jesus' healing. Nowhere in the Bible can you find the words, "Healing is only for the people of this time." It was for people back then, and it is still for people today.

I look at it this way: If healing isn't for today, then salvation isn't for today either. And if salvation isn't for today and the teachings in the Bible aren't for today, then why not throw away your Bible? Just trash it. Or if you're into antiques, put it on the shelf with other ancient books that don't do anything.

I know that is a strong statement, but the Bible tells us in Isaiah 55:11 that the Word of God will *not* return void:

> **So shall my word be that goeth forth out of my mouth: it shall not return unto me void, but it shall accomplish that which I please, and it shall prosper in the thing whereto I sent it.**

By saying that healing is not for today, people are literally saying that God's Word *does* stop working somewhere along the way. That is inaccurate if you consider Isaiah's prophetic words. Of course, you can go to heaven regardless of whether you believe that Jesus can heal or not. Acceptance of Jesus as Lord is all it takes to get through the pearly gates. But why suffer when Jesus already suffered for you? Why suffer when He so compassionately gave Himself to be beaten for your sake?

God isn't cutting out sections and chapters of the Bible. He is not saying, "Well, Peter could use this part, but you can't." That would make Him a respecter of persons, and Romans 2:11 sets the record straight when it says, **For there is no respect of persons with God.**

Jesus Is Still Anointed, Compassionate and Dedicated To Recognizing Faith

When Jesus was on the earth, He demonstrated His will to heal many, many times. Matthew 4:23-25 shows that:

> And Jesus went about all Galilee, teaching in their synagogues, and preaching the gospel of the kingdom, and healing all manner of sickness and all manner of disease among the people.
>
> And his fame went throughout all Syria: and they brought unto him all sick people that were taken with divers diseases and torments, and those which were possessed with devils, and those which were lunatick, and those that had the palsy; and he healed them. And there followed him great multitudes of people from Galilee, and from Decapolis, and from Jerusalem, and from Judaea, and from beyond Jordan.

Jesus was in the business of teaching, preaching, making disciples, healing sick people and running off demons. In the Great Commission in Mark 16:17,18 it says,

> And these signs shall follow them that believe; in my name shall they cast out devils; they shall speak with new tongues; they shall take up serpents; and if they drink any deadly thing, it shall not hurt them; they shall lay hands on the sick, and they shall recover.

You see, Jesus expected His disciples to carry on with His work.

Jesus did all of the things He mentioned in these verses. And it wasn't something He did every once in awhile; it was His lifestyle. He didn't go around healing people just to show them that He was God either. He demonstrated the power of healing because 1) He was anointed to heal, 2) He had compassion on the sick and 3) He recognized people's faith.

Today, Jesus is still anointed. He still has compassion. And He still recognizes faith. He has promised to extend His healing blood to us when we believe Him.

Jesus Is Willing

Another passage about Jesus' willingness to heal can be found in Mark 1:40-41 NIV. In this story we learn about the difference between Jesus' being able to heal, and Jesus' being willing to heal. A leper fell at Jesus' feet and said, **"If You are willing, You can make me clean."** The Bible says that Jesus was moved with compassion, stretched out His hand and touched the man. He said, **"I am willing...be cleansed."** Through this we learn that Jesus is willing to heal people.

Now, Jesus could have said, "Yeah, I can—but I won't!" He could have said, "I'm not touching you; you're contagious, and I don't want to get what you've got!" But He didn't. Again He was 1) anointed to heal, 2) moved with compassion and 3) He recognized the man's faith in Him. Jesus was willing to heal the leper, and He is willing to heal you.

All Scripture Is Given to You!

I know that there are some people who really get shook up when I use certain Scriptures in the Bible. When I say that they can stand on the same ones, they worry and think, *That Scripture isn't for me. Jesus was talking to His disciples.* Or they think, *Paul said that when he was writing to that Theo guy; it isn't really meant for me.*

You may have read John 15:1-12, where Jesus tells His disciples He is the true vine and they are the branches—and said to yourself, *Really though, wasn't that just to the people of that day? Does that really apply to me? After all, Jesus said it over 2000 years ago to people who are dead and gone! How can that apply to me?*

If you've ever thought any of these things, allow me to let you in on a truth. When Jesus was speaking there to His disciples, He *wasn't* just speaking to them. He was actually speaking to you and me today. But not just to you and me. He was speaking to our ancestors and our children, to generations in the past, present and future. How do I know that? Because of 2 Timothy 3:16-17.

There it says,

All Scripture is given by inspiration of God, and is profitable for doctrine, for reproof, for correction, for instruction in righteousness: that the man of God may be perfect, thoroughly furnished unto all good works.

That's the *King James Version,* and it is considered one of the more accurate versions we've got today.

The *New International Version* puts it another way. It states,

All Scripture is God-breathed and is useful for teaching, rebuking, correcting and training in righteousness, so that the man of God may be thoroughly equipped for every good work.

The *New American Standard Bible* says it this way,

All Scripture is inspired by God and profitable for teaching, for reproof, for correction, for training in righteousness;

so that the man of God may be adequate, equipped for every good work.

The Amplified Bible goes even further. It says,

Every Scripture is God-breathed–given by His inspiration–and profitable for instruction, for reproof and conviction of sin, for correction of error and discipline in obedience, and for training in righteousness [that is, in holy living, in conformity to God's will in thought, purpose and action], so that the man of God may be complete and proficient, well-fitted and thoroughly equipped for every good work.

As you can see, no matter what the version, the message is crystal clear: The Word of God *is* for you and me today. Hebrews 13:8 even further confirms this truth when it says, **Jesus Christ the same yesterday, and to day, and for ever.**

Jesus' teachings *are* for you, and don't let anybody talk you out of that with a bunch of logistics and theology. That religious stuff will choke the life right out of you! The theological wilderness has no soft grass or refreshing water of the Word. It is nothing but thickets and thorns and a royal pain in the you-know-what to try to live by.

Jesus, on the other hand, cut through all of that mess. His words were like a big sickle, slicing through the hypocrisy and making more room for the truth.

Jesus Knew How To Cut Through the Crud

Jesus had a really good habit of "cutting through the crud." Religious hypocrisy didn't get an ounce of slack from Him. Jesus

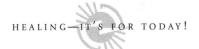

boiled it all down to the issues of the human heart and would lash out at those who sought to choke the heart of the issues with hypocritical rules.

When in Mark 7, for example, the religious scholars criticized Jesus for not washing His hands before He ate, He lashed out at them for being so ridiculously strict about washing the outside while their insides remained a vile place of filth. Oh, they didn't like that one bit! Can you imagine people looking at you in disgust because you forgot to wash your hands and then your retaliating at them by saying, "Look, I may not have washed my hands, but my heart is pure while you're full of all sorts of filthy trash!" Or, "You may look good on the outside, but you're just whitewashed tombs full of nothing but stinkin', rotting bones, you filthy Pharisees!"

Jesus Wasn't a Wimp

Jesus wasn't a wimp. He wasn't some mealy-mouthed preacher who walked around in a daze all the time, disconnected from the outside world. He didn't take as much junk off people as you might think. Unless He was being persecuted for God's sake, He didn't let people beat on Him. He'd either say something or walk away.

One time in the temple Jesus got so hot under the collar that He started making a rope! In other words, He was considering beating the tar out of something! He drove the merchants right off the temple grounds, turning over their tables and hollering at them! He said they'd made the church a den of thieves. (John 2:13-17.) He was right. He got to the heart of the issue, and people understood really quickly what He meant!

Jesus was wise. He sought to help people live purely both in their hearts and in their actions. He wanted to clean out the old ideas that man had hung on the Bible and get back to the truth of what God said. Go ahead and reread the gospels of Matthew, Mark, Luke and John for yourself. Read what Jesus had to say when situations arose, and you'll see that time after time, He talked about the heart of the matter.

Jesus showed us that God could and would do miracles of salvation, healing, deliverance and even prosperity if we would only believe. Phrases like "Be it according to your faith" and "Your faith hath made you whole" are throughout the Gospels. In other words, what is in your heart? Is it belief and trust in God that dominates? Or is it doubt and skepticism?

It's What Is in Your Heart That Matters

It's what is in your heart that matters. It's what you *do* with what God gives you that makes the difference in receiving your healing or not.

You may say, "How do I get off of drugs? How do I get healed? How do I get all of these things out of my life?" The answer is by breaking the power of natural law in your own life. Nobody can do it for you. Even though God may use others to stimulate your faith in Him and pray the prayer of agreement with you, ultimately it is *your* faith that will make you whole spirit, soul and body.

Say this to yourself: "My success doesn't depend on how much of the Word I read or know about; it depends on how much of the Word I allow to become a part of me." I'm not just talking about applying the Word here, but I'm talking about becoming *one* with it—abiding in it.

Unite yourself with the Word in the same way you united yourself with Jesus when you accepted Him as your Savior. Can you do that? Say, "Yes, I can," even if you're unsure right now. I believe that as you start sowing the Word into your mind, you'll begin to have confidence and build faith. Your heart will be opened to believe more. Your childlike faith will begin to flower, and natural law will begin to break.

I've seen many, many people succeed in breaking the power of natural law in their lives. I've had it happen to me, and I know without a shadow of doubt that it can happen to *you*. Now that we've laid the some foundation on salvation, faith and God's will concerning healing, let's get into some serious natural law-breaking Scripture. Let's dive into the red-hot truth of John 15. I just love it when Jesus starts talking in red!

The Red-Hot Truth of John 15

on't you love the red parts of the Bible? Those red parts are smoking with power! In John 15:1, Jesus starts off with two little red words that I just love. He begins, **I am....** You may not think much of those two words, but when I hear them they remind me of Exodus 3:13-14.

And Moses said unto God, Behold, when I come unto the children of Israel, and shall say unto them, The God of your fathers hath sent me unto you; and they shall say to me, What is his name? what shall I say unto them? [Moses wanted to know what God's name was.] **And God said unto Moses, I AM THAT I AM: and he said, Thus shalt thou say unto the children of Israel, I AM hath sent me unto you.**

When God responded, "I AM THAT I AM," Moses got a revelation! There just isn't a name big enough to house the Almighty God! Yahweh! Elohim! Jehovah! Healer! Provider! Comforter! Counselor! None can match up to Him. He is who He is. And that is that!

Verse 1—Jesus Is the Real Deal

In chapter 2 of this book, we established the singularity of Jesus as the true vine by looking at the red-hot words of Jesus Himself: **I am the true vine, and my Father is the husbandman** (John 15:1).

Verse 2—Your Mission in Life Is To Bear Some Fruit

Every branch in me that beareth not fruit he taketh away: and every branch that beareth fruit, he purgeth it, that it may bring forth more fruit.

JOHN 15:2

If you're hooked up to the vine by way of salvation, then your job is to bear some fruit. But what is Jesus talking about when He tells us to bear fruit?

Jesus is talking about inner attributes. From those inner attributes comes a change in our heart which then turns into a change in our lifestyle and an urge to do good. Galatians 5:22-23 lists these inner attributes and calls them the fruit of the Spirit.

The fruit of the Spirit is *love, joy, peace, longsuffering, gentleness, goodness, faith, meekness, temperance:* **against such there is no law.**

It goes on to say in verses 24 and 25, **And they that are Christ's have crucified the flesh with the affections and lusts. If we live in the Spirit, let us also walk in the Spirit.**

Throughout the Bible you can find Scriptures that compare our lives to a fruit-bearing branch, vine or tree. Again, our biblical forefathers were from an agricultural society. But even if you don't know a thing about agriculture, you can look outside and see for yourself the effects of tending trees and plants.

Those which are planted in good ground and are tended by pruning, or purging, grow well. Those that aren't—well, they struggle. And often they wither up and die. Then one day somebody comes along and pulls the dead things up from the root.

No Fruit or *Much* Fruit?

To the Lord, there are only two alternatives in fruit bearing. There is no such thing as little fruit. It is either 1) no fruit or 2) much fruit. And it is when you bear much fruit that He is glorified. Revelation 3:15-16 puts it this way: **I know thy works, that thou art neither cold nor hot: I would thou wert cold or hot. So then because thou art lukewarm, and neither cold nor hot, I will spue thee out of my mouth.**

Does that sound like an in-between God to you? No fruit or much fruit. Hot or cold. With God, it is either one way or the other. It is black or white. You believe the Bible, or you don't. There is no such thing as being "sort of saved" or "sort of healed." Either you are, or you aren't. Let's just be honest; fruit is either coming forth in your life, or it isn't. There isn't a mystery to why things happen. It is what you do that counts—not just what you believe. It is by your fruit that you know if you are a disciple of Jesus Christ. There is no such thing as little fruit.

Verse 3—The Soul-Scrubbing Action of the Word

In verse 3 of John 15, Jesus says, **Now ye are clean through the word which I have spoken unto you.**

According to this verse, you can't get clean by religion on its own. You can hear sermons until you're blue in the face. Regardless of how many times you go to church and kneel at the altar, if you do not believe the Word of God for yourself *personally*, getting clean is a pretty hard thing to do.

You could consider the Word your personal soul scrubber. If you don't take it and allow it to touch you personally, then it can't do a whole lot of good. It is like a Brillo pad left in a soap dish by the sink. The pad is a powerful cleaning tool, and it will work if you pick it up and move it across the surface of the sink. But if you never take it out of the dish, the sink won't get clean—no matter how many years the pad has been sitting there by the sink!

If you go to church and hear the Word but never take it for yourself personally, it's just religion. It's just a Brillo pad by the sink! It may soothe your conscience to attend the service, but it won't really help you to the degree that you need to see change. It won't help you produce fruit.

Getting clean doesn't come by personal experience either. I believe that you can lie on a couch in a therapist's office and spill the beans until you've got nothing left to tell. You can tell a friend all the trials and tribulations that you've been through in life. You can say, "Ohhhhh!" and "Ahhhhhh!" and "Didn't they do me wrong!" and "I'm so sick and tired of being sick and tired!" and "Just listen to what is going on in my life!" And all that might make you feel better, simply because you got it off your chest.

Your friend might say, "Do you know what I think you ought to do?" and give you some advice that you think is good enough to follow. But unless you put what is of *real* value—God's Word—into your heart and mind, you aren't going to be able to get really clean of the situation. You won't be able to tap into the peace you need. You won't be able to experience or share the fruit of love, joy, peace, longsuffering, gentleness, goodness, faith, meekness or temperance.

Let's face it, life can add all sorts of mess to your heart and mind. Only the living Word of God can clean that mess up. Only the Word of the living God can do what Psalm 51:10 says: **Create in me a clean heart, O God; and renew a right spirit within me.** You can't create the fruit of the Spirit on your own. It only comes by way of a relationship with God and a heart that allows His Word to change you.

God has some good advice. It's better than anybody else's advice. In fact, He has a book full of advice that would put the highest paid shrink on the map out of business. Those red words aren't just salve over the cuts and scrapes. They aren't Band-Aids that cover the wounds life has put on you.

God's Word is a real healing agent. When you take His advice and receive the healing power of His Word in your heart, you will be made clean. And it can happen in an instant. The moment you open your heart and expose that problem, whatever it is, to God's healing touch, you create an atmosphere to break natural law. In that moment God's Word and your trust in Him to perform it collide, and His healing power comes suddenly.

Verse 4—How Do You Bear Fruit?

Jesus says in verse 4, **Abide in me, and I in you. As the branch cannot bear fruit of itself, except it abide in the vine; no more can ye, except ye abide in me.**

This Scripture compares fruit bearing to your life as a Christian. A vine can't produce a grape without being a part of the bigger main vine that's rooted in the ground. Likewise, you can't produce any real fruit in your life if you're not grounded in Jesus. Only by abiding in Him can you produce good fruit.

The word *abide* is similar to the words *dwell* and *inhabit*. It means to dwell in His presence or to make Jesus a part of your everyday life. I don't mean just a Sunday relationship with Jesus. I'm talking about an everyday thing! But what if we go beyond that? How about every *moment*?

Now, don't misunderstand me. I'm not talking about walking around in the clouds all day. It's not deep intercession twenty-four hours a day, seven days a week. Although that would be great, we've got to live in this world as lights in a dark place. If we're never really "here," then we're not illuminating anything.

To me, abiding simply means having a moment-to-moment awareness of God in my everyday life. It's as easy as recognizing Him and not ignoring Him. It's about being open to His voice and tuning in to the Holy Spirit within me.

In this verse Jesus assures you that if you treat Him this way, He will be sure to return the gesture. If you abide in Him, He will abide in you. If you choose to dwell in His presence, He will dwell in yours. If you don't want Him to abide with you, He won't! In other words, Jesus is a gentleman. He won't push Himself on you. But He will meet you right where you are—regardless of where that is.

Cooking With No Gas

In my ministry meetings, I often move heavily in the gifts of the Spirit. Often the Lord will quicken certain physical needs to me and prompt me to call those needs out so that people may come up and receive healing prayer.

Other times He will give me a word of knowledge for particular people within the congregation. I give the word; they receive it for themselves and often fall to the ground under the power of God. I don't push anybody down. I don't try to make it happen. If they cry, fine. If they don't, fine. If they fall, fine. If they don't, fine.

It's not my job to tug at anybody's emotions or try to play God by pushing people to the floor. If God wants to lay them out, He is more than welcome to do it without my giving a little push.

That is why it is so funny to me when people ask me to give a word to them or a friend. I've even had ministers ask me, "Brother Jesse, why don't you just give that person a word?" I think, *You've got to be kidding! You're a preacher! Don't you know that's not how it works?*

Some do know. But instead of pulling back when God isn't moving that way, they go ahead and say something to someone anyway. They give a "word from God" that is no more than good-sounding words. I call that cooking with no gas. No gas is coming through the fuel line. God hasn't told them to do anything. Yet they're fired up and speaking words as if God is fueling them on. He isn't. And that is how a lot of preachers mess up and miss God. It is a crying shame when a person steers his life on a different course as a result of a false "word."

Of course, the preacher giving the word is as wrong as a three-dollar bill. But I think that most of the time a preacher does it because he feels pressured. He may be taking the burden of the ministry on his own shoulders, not wanting to disappoint the people with a "bland" service. He may be worried about how the congregation views him, not wanting them to think that he is without God's power on his life. I know it sounds crazy, but let me tell you something—it happens.

If you're a preacher or a layperson who has been used of the Lord to give words of knowledge to others, I want you to know that you don't ever have to feel pressured to cook with no gas. You don't have to make it happen. That's what God is for.

No one falls down when you pray? So what! God hasn't given you a message for anybody? So what! Ask the people to bow their heads, pray for them as a group, dismiss and go home!

If you feel in your spirit that God wants to do something but nothing is happening, don't start moving in your own strength. Don't disengage from the gas line! Just ask everyone to pray as a group and intercede until the Lord starts moving in some way. God will show you what to do, and best of all, you'll be *in* His will rather than moving against it. You'll go home with a clear conscience, and nobody will leave damaged by an uncontrolled flame!

If people came to a meeting looking for words of prophecy and none flowed, they may be disappointed. If they came expecting to see people rolling on the floor laughing or draped over the altars crying and it didn't happen, they may be disappointed. They may feel that way, but if they do, what does that have to do with you? Nothing!

You are just a vessel. If God isn't moving in a particular way, remind yourself that God is in control and He can do whatever He wants to do. God is a multifaceted Being, and He moves in all sorts of mysterious ways. I can guarantee that if you're open to His voice, if you're abiding in Him and He is abiding in you, then you will see more than one of His many facets! Not every service will be alike!

Verse 5—Without God, You Can Do Nothing That Is Really Important

I am the vine, ye are the branches: He that abideth in me, and I in him, the same bringeth forth much fruit: for without me ye can do nothing.

JOHN 13:5

Notice Jesus said that He is the vine. *He* is the vine, not the branches. You're a branch, not the vine. He promised that if you abide in Him you'll bring forth much fruit. Not more fruit, but much fruit.

Then He went on to say that without Him, you can do nothing of any real importance or value. Some things may seem to be of importance, but in the long run they're not. Without Jesus involved in your life, your life is just filled with a bunch of occurrences that fall into the "nothing" category. As a preacher I know that it doesn't matter how well preachers speak. It doesn't matter how eloquent they are behind the pulpit. Without the anointing of Jesus on them, they're just babbling words that have no power.

If I didn't have any anointing, I could preach on salvation all day long, and a chicken wouldn't even come up and get saved! It is the anointing that breaks the yoke of bondage on people's lives.

(Isaiah 10:27.) It is the anointing of the Holy Spirit that draws them. Religion puts on a yoke of condemnation and guilt, but the Holy Spirit destroys that stuff! Glory!

I know that if I want my life to go in the right direction, I have to include God in my decision-making. When I want to make major decisions in my life or when I want to change directions, I immediately go to God. Sometimes He leads me by His still, small voice. Other times, He just gives me a peace about the situation. But there have been times when I've come to God with a situation, and instead of giving me His answer, He has let me use my own judgement.

Once I came to Him about a certain decision I had to make and asked, "What do you think about this?"

He spoke to my heart and said, *Whatever you decide will be fine.*

"Are you serious?" I asked.

Yeah! Fine. I trust you!

It was odd to have Him do that back then. Now He does it a lot. I find that the closer I get to Him, the more decisions He trusts me with. Of course, God knows that I'm not looking to make a decision that is against His will, which is His Word. I'm not saying, "Hey, how much can I skirt around this thing? How much can I get away with?" No, I love God, and I want to do right. I remember as much Word as I can and make sure to do His will. By not going against His Word, I know I'm making the best decision.

You've heard people ask, "What would Jesus do?" Answer that, and you've got the best decision. But if you don't know Him or His

Word, you can't really answer that question in all honesty. And that's where abiding comes in again.

If you're abiding and dwelling in Jesus, your judgement will be clear. You may already know in your heart the right decision. You may go to the Lord and hear Him tell you, *Whatever you decide will be fine.* I think it is a great honor to have the Lord show that kind of trust.

Verse 6—You Were Created To Thrive, Not Whither

If a man abide not in me, he is cast forth as a branch, and is withered.... Not only is he cut out, he is withered, or crippled. **...And men gather them, and cast them into the fire, and they are burned** (v. 6). Now, this is pretty clear-cut. If you don't make Christ your home—if you're not connected to the true vine—you're in the spiritually crippling process of withering. And soon enough men will try to burn you to nothing and obliterate you. Notice that *men* will do this, not God.

My wife, Cathy, kills plants. She's merciless. The woman can flat kill a plant. Or if she doesn't kill it, she brings it to the very brink of death, and then suddenly she lavishes attention on it. Plants don't know what to do in our house. They never know where their next drink is coming from.

We get these plants because sometimes people send them to us as gifts. I feel sorry for the plants when I see them come in the door, all shiny and full. I say, "You're about to bite the dust, plant. That's it. Your glory days are over. Welcome to Cathy's house." Sure enough, a week or so goes by, and they start sulking in their pots. I can hear their dry, weakened little voices saying, "I'll tell you one thing, I wish that woman would water us." Their little branches are hanging halfway off the edge of the pot. They've lost some leaves already, and they're holding on for life.

Cathy says our plants die because we travel so much and she just can't keep up with them. Or she says I'm exaggerating, which I'm not. They're thirsty. I can see it. They're parched and dry and begging for a drop of water. "Please, Mr. Jesse, a little water?" they say when I walk by them. I give them a swig from my glass and say, "Here you go, plant."

I tell Cathy that she should get rid of them or give them to somebody who won't torture them. It's sad. We need plastic at our house. Green plastic. That's what my wife can keep alive.

Cathy used to keep plants on the brink of death like that all the time. They'd be just about gone, and suddenly she'd get the hankering to start caring for them like babies. She'd water them and give them some kind of blue fertilizer stuff. She'd start tending to them and clipping their dead leaves off. They'd perk up, and things would really be going great. For a couple of weeks or so this would go on, and the plants would say, "Hey, this is good! Things are good!" And then back to the torture chambers.

No water. No food. No light. They'd start drooping and hanging over the pot again.

Nowadays she gives them to Jodi, our daughter, and her husband, Ed. Over at their house, it's not quite as bad. But the girl has a little of her mother's black thumb, so sometimes it's almost the same thing. Some live; some die. But at least I don't have to watch it happen. Let Ed pick up the dead leaves.

A lot of Christians treat their spirits the same way my wife treats plants. They let themselves get so parched and dry until they're barely alive. They don't feed their spirits the milk of the Word, much less the meat.

Those Christians are like plants that go long stretches of time with no fertilizer, no water and no sunlight. They go for long periods of time with no studying of the Word, no applying of the Word and no time in the presence of God. What do you think happens to a person under those conditions? Yeah, you've got it. The same thing that happens to Cathy's plants. They start to wither. Then they dry up completely. And given enough time without the things they need to live, they'll die. Then what happens? Men come to throw them out. Can you guess who that is in my house? Yeah, me. My job is taking out the trash—getting rid of what can't be used. Are you getting the comparison here?

Jesus told us that we need to take care of our spiritual selves. If we continually neglect Jesus and His teachings, we'll begin to wither. The peace that comes from spending time with Jesus slips right out the window. The strength that comes from the joy of the Lord goes too. Then we're weak and full of anxiety. That's not exactly a good place to be when life is throwing the punches.

You and I were never created to be hanging over the edge of a pot! We weren't created to be gasping for air and begging for a drop of water like a dying plant. We were created to thrive and grow to be mature, fruit-producing limbs of God's family tree. And how do we do that? By abiding in the One who gives us eternal life.

Verse 7—There Is a Condition To Asking for Something From God

Jesus said, **If ye abide in me, and my words abide in you, ye shall ask what ye will, and it shall be done unto you** (John 15:7). Here he gives us the secret to receiving our hearts' desires.

Now, reread this verse, and think of what you would ask. Do not limit Jesus. Do not limit this verse on behalf of religious ideas. It is written in red! Jesus meant what He said! He loves you and wants to do good for you.

I don't care how much religious experience you've had, right or wrong. You can't limit what God says, because He is limitless. He says that if you dwell in His presence and His Word dwells in your heart, you can ask what you will and it shall be done for you.

What do you *will*? What would you ask? Now, most importantly, would you be willing to follow the condition? What is the condition? It's that you dwell in His presence and His Word dwells in your heart. That is the condition, and only when you're doing this can you ask what you will and see it done for you.

So if you're not willing to dwell in His presence and have His Word dwell in your heart, then what? You can't really expect to ask God for something and see it done, can you? Now, that is strong, but it's what Jesus said. There is a condition here. Think on this Scripture, and ask yourself what you're really willing to do.

This is a great verse that lets us know our part in receiving from God. Yet it is overlooked so often. Why? Because it requires something. It requires a communicating relationship with the Lord. It requires the Word of God to be a part of your life.

Verse 8—Glorify God! Be His Disciple! Bear Much Fruit!

Herein is my Father glorified, that ye bear much fruit; so shall ye be my disciples.

JOHN 15:8

When you fulfill these verses in John 15, God is glorified.

When you recognize His Son as the true vine, God is glorified.

When you accept your place as a branch on God's family tree, God is glorified.

When you bear much fruit in your life, God is glorified.

When you abide in Him, God is glorified.

When His Word abides in you, God is glorified.

When you ask what you will, God is glorified.

When He does it for you, God is glorified.

Then, God says, when these things have happened you have become a disciple of Jesus. It is by your *fruit* that you are seen by Him and by others as His disciple. Only by your fruit can you be known as a disciple of Christ.

The inner attributes of love, joy, peace, longsuffering, gentleness, goodness, faith, meekness, temperance and the good works you do because these things are flowing in your life prove that you are a disciple of Jesus Christ.

I think of my fruit as how I think, what I do and how I act. If I am a good witness for Jesus, if I speak the Word and people come to the knowledge of Christ as a result, then I am bearing good fruit and glorifying my Father in heaven.

To me, souls won for the kingdom are the number-one sign of good fruit. I'm dedicated to this evangelistic ministry. It is my life. It is what I live for. I believe that telling others about Jesus or showing others how to get the most out of their relationship with God proves that I've got love in my heart for other people.

But I also think that just spreading the joy of the Lord to others is bearing fruit too. If I have patience with my wife, I get excited! Why? Because I'm bearing fruit! If I am gentle with someone and don't tear him down on account of a weakness he might have, then I'm bearing fruit! Whatever I do that is good, whatever I say or think that is good, I consider to be the fruit of my life.

The fruit of the Spirit Galatians 5:22-23 talks about could be considered attributes of your maker, God. And without His presence in your life, you can't get them. You could try to fake love, joy, peace and so forth. But without God, those fruits of the Spirit can't really exist in your life.

Only the Lord can produce fruit in your life. Only you can draw close enough to Him and put His Word in your heart to receive them. When you have the fruit of the Spirit in your life, good works will flow from you freely. People will know you by your fruit. How can you tell you're bearing fruit?

When you show love to yourself and others, you are bearing fruit.

When you are joyful and spread joy to others, you are bearing fruit.

When you are longsuffering, or patient, with yourself and others, you are bearing fruit.

When you act gently with yourself and others, you are bearing fruit.

When you "do good," "think good" and "talk good" about yourself and others, you are bearing fruit.

When you have faith in God and in His ability and will to perform His Word, you are bearing fruit.

God is glorified when you choose not to limit Him and not to limit yourself. You can do all things through Christ who strengthens you. (Philippians 4:13.) You can have the fruit of the Spirit working in your life. You can do good works and live your life with a clean conscience, knowing that you are living your life as God would have you live it. And how is that? In love.

Only That Which Bears the Stamp of Eternity Can Really Be Called Fruit

When God sent Jesus to the earth, He expected a harvest—a body of believers called Christians—to come out of the seed sown called Christ. Jesus was God's seed. Christ was sowed, and Christians are continuing to be harvested. You and I are the very fruit of God, and our lives should be dedicated to sowing our witness within the earth.

Whatever you sow on this earth will follow you into eternity after your death. The fruit of the Spirit is eternal. The fruit that you produce and allow to flow in your life is pure and is the only thing that can rightly be called fruit. All the good that you think, say and do in this life will follow you into eternity. God will thank you for it during that great Judgement Day. He will bring to account your fruit in this life. He'll show you when you did right and when you missed it. When that day comes you'll see it all from God's perspective—the strength or lack of faith, the positive or negative thoughts and words, the little or much fruit bearing in your life.

What you pass on to others in this earth is what really matters, because only what bears the stamp of eternity can be called fruit.

Have you heard about sowing and reaping? Sure you have. But that doesn't just have to do with finances. I believe it has to do with everything in life. Your very life is a seed. What you put in the ground will come up. If you put what is good in the ground, you'll see that good come up. If you sow what is bad, you'll see that come up too.

I am a giver, and I've had people ask me, "Brother Jesse, why do you give so much?" My answer is pretty simple. First, I like to give. It's so much fun. It's a blessing, and it is the nature of God who lives *in* me. God is a giver, so I am too. Secondly, I know that the only thing I'm going to take to heaven is what I give away. That is what I'll be judged for. I pay attention to how much seed I've got in the ground because that is what is going to be talked about up there.

How many people did I witness to? How many people did I bless with joy? How many churches did I help become debt-free?

How many people received Jesus because the church was able to spend its money on more evangelism? How many kids did I send to Bible school to learn the oracles of God? How many heard my testimony of deliverance? How many heard the Word of faith and healing? How many people did I get to lay hands on and pray for? How many were changed because of the Word of God abiding in my life? How many words did I preach that changed people's lives? How much of myself did I give away?

These are the types of questions I ask myself when I consider my own fruit. It's not about me, me and me. It is about others, others and more others. Good fruit bearing is what is most important in life. Touching the lives of others with whatever the Lord gave you is what it is all about.

God gave me a gift. He gave me a calling too. He expects me to use that gift and talents I have to help others grow and produce fruit of their own. In the world, people could care less about one another. They're out for their four and no more. But with God, it is different. Although His church is made up of human, fallible beings, we still should be doing more than the world. We should care more, do more and talk more about changing this world to be a better place than any other group of people. It is our moral responsibility to bear good fruit.

I'm not saying you have to be perfect; I'm just saying you have to care. This Christianity is a gospel of love and caring for mankind. It is a gospel of truth that cares enough about other people to let them know, "Hey, I know a better way. Let me tell you what Jesus is all about."

Verse 9—Love: The Mark of God's Hand on Your Life

As the Father hath loved me, so have I loved you; continue ye in my love

JOHN 15:9

Continue is an action word. We ought to show love to other people and continue to do it throughout our lives. Through our words and our actions, love is the mark of God's hand on our lives. It shows with whom we keep company.

Notice that Jesus didn't make a distinction between the love of God and you. So don't let religious people get you down in the dumps by spreading their condemnation on you; no matter what you do, God loves you just as He loves Jesus. Think about that!

There is no distinction between God's loving Jesus and Jesus' loving you. It's all the same love, flowing from the throne of God, going through Jesus, into you and out from you to others. Those others then turn to God and give back the love that He began. That's how love continues to flow on the earth. Jesus said that! It's written in red, so you know it's the truth!

Love changes things on the earth. Why? Because it is connected to God. There is no other source that love can come from but Him. First John 4:8 says that God *is* love. Love is not just a part of Him, it literally is Him! This is why He commands us, **Continue ye in my love** (John 15:9). We must keep His love flowing to others in this earth.

Love is your calling in life. It's my calling in life. It was Jesus' calling in life too.

Galatians 5:19-21 tells us what types of bad fruit come when a person *doesn't* abide in God. It shows what the flip side to the fruit of the Spirit is. They are called the works of the flesh and can be considered bad fruit:

> **Now the works of the flesh are manifest, which are these; adultery, fornication, uncleanness, lasciviousness, idolatry, witchcraft, hatred, variance, emulations, wrath, strife, seditions, heresies, envyings, murders, drunkenness, revellings, and such like: of the which I tell you before, as I have also told you in time past, that they which do such things shall not inherit the kingdom of God.**

Of course, you may not go so far as to do all of these, but even if one has a foothold in your life, it shows that what you're abiding in isn't producing good fruit in your life.

After all, if we're bitter and angry, we're bearing bad fruit. If we're envious and full of jealousy, we're bearing bad fruit. If we steal, kill or destroy, we're bearing bad fruit. If we gossip and hurt others with our words and our actions, we're bearing bad fruit. All of those seemingly harmless actions are pieces of rancid fruit.

Have you ever seen a Christian bashing another person with words? Or how about one doing that in the name of God? Maybe you've seen them on TV, picketing and hollering hate-driven words at sinners. I can't stand it when I see so-called Christians on TV hollering hate-filled words at sinners. To me, even if the other person is wrong and in sin, how is he or she ever going to be won to Christ through words of hate? They are just tearing sinners to shreds and giving them no hope. That isn't love; it is hate cloaked in religion.

This Gospel is a gospel of love. That doesn't mean that it is a passive gospel that allows any old, sinful thing to happen in the name of love, but it does mean that our words and actions should be motivated by the love of God.

Lemons and Persimmons

I try to examine myself for fruit. I ask the Lord, "Is my fruit growing, Jesus?" I try to taste some of my own fruit to see if it is sweet or sour. I don't want to be a lemon, you know! I don't want to be a persimmon! Lemons and persimmons look beautiful until you bite into them.

There are some Christians like that. They're bearing lemon fruit and persimmon fruit. You get close to them and get a bite of their fruit. Oh, your face contorts, and all you want to do is wince and spit! Do you know people like that?

You know you're a lemon when people try to avoid you. Check your fruit! Maybe you're passing around so much lemon juice that people are running for cover. People who put off sweet fruit are more attractive than people who put off bitter-tasting fruit.

When I first got saved I was a long-haired hippie freak, to use the vernacular of that time. I remember walking into a church and hearing a guy say, "You won't last long with that hair on your head." I was going to church looking for sweet-tasting fruit, but what I got was a shot of lemon juice! The stuff hit me in the face, and before I knew what to do, I was wincing and spitting.

Here's another example. When the "fruit of the womb" first comes on the scene, it is not much sweetness either. When my daughter was born, she didn't come out to meet a world of sweetness. She went through a tough time just getting out, and then she was met with a slap!

Whack! Welcome to the world, kid! My daughter didn't come out fully clothed either. She came out hungry, screaming and naked!

I imagine that Jodi was sleeping before that time, warm and happy in the womb. Then came the contractions. Her little head was being squeezed and beaten around. Then imagine this—a big pair of metal forceps came at her, trying to grab on to her skull and yank her out. *Whew!* It's rough! I think that is why God doesn't let us remember it. Who'd want to?

I didn't feel too sorry for her, though, because I had it worse. I came out with a veil over my face! At least Jodi could see! I came out of the womb with a thin covering of skin over my face. They called babies like me "veil babies" back then. So I got slapped on the rear and then cut on the face! *Welcome to the world, Jesse! People are going to cut you for the rest of your life. Get used to it.* The doctor looked at me and thought, *You're worth a fat fee to me, little man, and a little extra with that veil.*

I had a stamp when I came out of the womb—"Duplantis." God took it even further when I accepted Him into my life. He stamped me "a son of God." He spoke the Word and inspired men to write it down so that I could live up to my stamp. You were stamped too—"a daughter of God" or "a son of God." The Word of God is here to help you live up to your stamp.

Now that you're a Christian, the fruit of the Spirit is what is in you. Your Father is God, and what is in Him is what you should be producing. Lemons don't come from pineapple fields. Persimmons don't grow from orange trees.

Because you are living your life abiding in God, the people you communicate with are going to find that they can draw out divine energy from you. As you abide, you'll find that others will eat from the sweet fruit you produce. You won't be sustaining them—God will—but He will use you! Jesus will give you the strength to produce sweet, fulfilling fruit for those who desperately need a refreshing. If you're the one who needs a refreshing, there are people who will be producing fruit for you to partake of.

All of the Bible's Teachings Are Connected

You may ask, "But why is this important for me personally? What does it have to do with breaking natural law?" Well, for one thing, you've got to understand that all of the Bible's teachings are connected. They come from the same God. And if you are having a really hard time receiving something like healing or deliverance, it's time to go through that Word and see what makes what click. It's time to check other things in your life that may be hindering your ability to receive.

Take faith, for instance. Although there are a lot of Scriptures that reflect on faith, there is one that lets us in on a little secret, one Scripture that shows us how faith works. It's in Galations 5:6, and it says, **For in Jesus Christ neither circumcision availeth any thing, nor uncircumcision;** *but faith which worketh by love.*

You see, there are a lot of people today running around trying to use faith to move the hand of God, but they don't have an ounce of love working in their lives. They may have pent-up anger and resentment toward a certain person. They may be deceitful in the way they go about things. They may be actually hindering their own faith by not walking in love, not spreading joy, not being longsuffering or acting gently, and not doing, saying or thinking good. They wonder, *Why isn't this faith stuff working?* I say, "Check your love." Most importantly, check your heart! All that stuff clogs up faith. It hinders a person from moving forward.

Faith Is Activated by Love

Love is the prerequisite to faith. And I know that without faith, it is not only impossible to please God, but it is also impossible to break natural law. (Hebrews 11:6.) It takes faith in God to break natural law and receive something like healing. It takes love to activate faith.

Go to God So He Can Clean Your Act Up

So make sure you're walking in love. In fact, go to God so He can clean your act up. Don't misunderstand me. You don't have to clean your act up before you go to God. It's the other way around. You've got to go to God so that *He* can clean your act up! And He'll clean you up as fast as you'll allow Him to. As much area as you give Him in which to abide, He'll wash clean with His blood. God will meet you where you are, wherever that may be. But He is a gentleman and won't go any further than you allow.

This is why being childlike and open before God is so important in breaking the power of natural law. When you're open before Him, He'll come right in and clean out all the stuff that is holding you back. Check your heart for what you consider "off limits" to God. Make sure there is nothing in there that is clogging up your childlike faith.

Verse 10—Keep Jesus' Commandments And You Will Automatically Abide in Love

If ye keep my commandments, ye shall abide in my love; even as I have kept my Father's commandments and abide in His love.

JOHN 15:10

Jesus gives a condition when He says, "If you keep My commandments...." If you do that, then you reap the reward: "...you will abide in My love." He gives you an example of Himself by saying, "I keep My Father's commandments, so I abide in His love." In other words, He is not asking you to do anything that He isn't doing. And He wouldn't tell you to do it if you weren't able to accomplish it.

So what are Jesus' commandments? Remember the Golden Rule—"Do unto others as you would have them do to you"? Here are the Scriptures that we derive it from:

First, in Leviticus 19:18: **Thou shalt not avenge, nor bear any grudge against the children of thy people,** *but thou shalt love thy neighbour as thyself:* **I am the Lord.**

Then in Matthew 7:12: *Therefore all things whatsoever ye would that men should do to you, do ye even so to them:* for this is the law and the prophets.

Again in Luke 6:31, *And as ye would that men should do to you, do ye also to them likewise.*

In Romans 13:9 it gets even more specific, outlining the Ten Commandments and ending with the Golden Rule: **For this, Thou shalt not commit adultery, Thou shalt not kill, Thou shalt not steal, Thou shalt not bear false witness, Thou shalt not covet; and if there be any other commandment, it is briefly comprehended in this saying, namely,** *Thou shalt love thy neighbour as thyself.*

And finally, in Galatians 5:14: **For all the law is fulfilled in one word, even in this;** *Thou shalt love thy neighbour as thyself.*

Jesus hit it on the nose in Matthew 7:12 when He said that all the law and the prophets are hinged on the Golden Rule. Everything falls into place when you do it. And isn't one rule pretty easy to remember?

Verse 11—You Can Be Full of Joy!

These things have I spoken unto you, that my joy might remain in you, and that your joy might be full.

JOHN 15:11

There are two kinds of joy spoken about in this verse: Jesus' joy and your joy. I like that Jesus says He told us these things so His joy could *remain* in us. I don't know about you, but I really do want Jesus' joy to remain in me! I don't want it to just hang around for a day or two; I want it to last my whole life. To me, that's what it means to be *full!*

Full, Remaining Joy Comes From the Inside, Not the Outside

Joy is one sought-after fruit. People are looking to be happy, and they'll do just about anything for some joy. Sadly, even Christians often think it's an unattainable thing. But joy isn't some mysterious gift from God. It isn't somewhere out there, waiting for you to find it. It doesn't come from other people or accomplishments in life. You can get some happiness from life, but lasting joy? No way!

Joy is a spiritual gift that doesn't come from the outside. It comes from the *inside.* Joy isn't around you, but it is literally *in* you. That is the miracle of the new birth. Consider that! The joy of the Lord is in you right now, regardless of how you feel. Because you are a believer, you can tap into it and watch it go to work for you.

Jesus knew that life would be tough sometimes. He knew we would go through tribulations in this sin-filled earth. And He told us what to do about tribulation. He said, **These things I have spoken unto you, that in me ye might have peace. In the world ye shall have tribulation: but be of good cheer; I have overcome the world** (John 16:33). In response to tribulation, Jesus commands us to draw on the spiritual fruit of joy. Our comfort comes from knowing that He has already overcome the world and all the tribulations that are in it. And as His kids, we're entitled to share in that victory.

Some people want God to dump joy on them first, and then they'll be of good cheer. But that is like putting the cart before the horse. The way to get down the road fast is to put the horse before the cart and let the horse do the hard work. Draw on the fruit of the Spirit dwelling in you first. How? By fulfilling His command to abide in Him and allowing His words to abide in you. The action of abiding is the horse that pulls the joy cart. It is where your power comes from.

When tribulation comes, I've seen a lot of people who actually back away from God. Then they wonder why they're so depressed. I always say, "If you want to be depressed, just stop talking to God. Skip church. Stop reading your Bible for awhile. Stop praising Him. Let the world wear on you a little, and sure enough, the devil will start throwing all kinds of depressing thoughts at you." He'll even throw in a little cynicism with your depression. Cynicism and depression—now, there is a bone-drying combination! Mix that with a tribulating circumstance, and you've got problems!

Now, I understand that it is hard to be happy when you're sick. It's hard to be happy when you're struggling with something or someone in your life. That's understandable. You are human. You are an emotional creature, and I understand that sometimes the flesh tries to take over. But I believe that joy is a *choice*. It is a spiritual choice that can change soulish emotions.

A Merry Heart Doeth Good Like a Medicine

God gave us a clue about the effect of joy on our bodies when He put Proverbs 17:22 in the Bible. There it says, **A merry heart doeth good like a medicine: but a broken spirit drieth the bones.** God said a merry or cheerful, joyful heart works like a medicine!

I think of joy like a prescription for my body. It is one of the active ingredients for my success. It isn't a filler, an optional fruit of the Spirit that I can do without. I know that if I want to live well, I've got to tap into the Source within me and take a dose of Holy Ghost joy.

I don't just do it because I'd rather be happy than sad. I do it because I know that it's a way for the healing power of God to flow through my mortal body. The joy of the Lord becomes my strength in every way. And with the kind of family medical history mine has, I know I've got to do whatever God says to stay strong!

Depression Is in Direct Opposition to Your Success in Breaking Natural Law

Now, if joy strengthens a person, then what does a broken, sad or grievous spirit do? It works the opposite way—it weakens a person. Like a bone-drying poison, a broken spirit makes you even more sick. So depression is in direct opposition to your success in breaking natural law in your life and receiving healing.

Now, don't misunderstand me. I'm not talking about feeling down sometimes. While we all have emotions, depression is the deep sorrow and grief that tries to get inside you and shut you down. That kind of sorrow is from the devil, and it's damaging.

Don't think Jesus doesn't know what you're going through. He does. Hebrews 4:15-16 lets us know,

> For we have not an high priest which cannot be touched with the feeling of our infirmities; but was in all points tempted like as we are, yet without sin. Let us therefore come boldly unto the throne of grace, that we may obtain mercy, and find grace to help in time of need.

Even Jesus Himself knew what it meant to be troubled by personal tribulation. Go back and read about His time in the Garden of Gethsemane if you don't believe me. He went to His Father in His time of need. (Luke 22:39-46.) But notice that Jesus didn't stay weeping in the garden forever. He got up and finished the work God had called Him to do. Thank God for that, because without Jesus' work on the Cross you wouldn't have a way out of grief and sorrow. Jesus made a way for you to be of good cheer when He overcame the world by way of the Cross! Isaiah 53:4 says, **Surely he hath borne our griefs, and carried our sorrows: yet we did esteem him stricken, smitten of God, and afflicted.**

Joy Is a Healing Force

Depression can be paralyzing. It can steal your joy and take away your normal ability to function. Just as joy is a healing force from God, depression is a sickening force from the devil. You can't mess with self-pity too long and not expect Satan to try to dump a load of bone-drying depression on you.

When Satan tries to hand me his spirit of brokenness, I have to make a conscious decision to stop myself from taking the road to sorrow and grief. When tribulation is hitting full force, I'll tell you, the easiest road to travel is the one that leads to depression. I know this. So I stop that idiot devil in his tracks. Why? Because boo-hooing never helped me out of one tribulation.

I have never felt any better dwelling on everything bad in my life. In fact, I've always felt worse. But when I resist the devil, do you know what he does? He flees! He has to. He has no other choice. (James 4:7.) And do you know what flees with him? All the garbage he has tried to hang on me, including depression and sadness. When I choose to refuse depression, when I choose to go to the throne of grace and tap into the fruit of the Spirit, the force of joy comes in and pushes the force of depression out.

Joy creates a change in my emotions. Suddenly my spirit starts telling my soul what to do! And you'd better know my emotions line up! Merriness makes its presence known, and that surge of joy creates a river of living water that starts to come out of my belly— my innermost being! Then I can pass it on to others who need a shot of joy.

We Give Our Natural Law-Breaking Power Away When We Confirm Satan's Lies

I heard a preacher say that we give our natural law-breaking power away when we confirm Satan's lies. That struck me as true. He said that the devil doesn't have any power on his own. We give him power when we confirm his lies. Why? Because *we* have power! We are made in the image of God! We are God's kids, powerful beings created by a powerful God, and our words mean something in this earth. So we lend power to whatever words we speak—good or evil.

This is a crucial truth when it comes to breaking the power of natural law. When we listen to God and choose His words, His power within us is released to flow and heal. When we listen to the devil and choose his deceiving words, we stop up the flow of healing. We actually give power to something Satan said. And that's dangerous.

Satan has no rightful power over your life. He may be able to hinder you by throwing his fiery darts of tribulation, but he doesn't have the power to stop you. Why? Because you are a blood-bought child of God. You're *literally* in God's family.

If you want to break the power of sin, sickness, addiction, financial trouble, relationship trouble or anything else that is hindering you from living an abundant life in Christ, you need to realize the power of agreeing with your Father God. You need to realize the importance of being connected to Him and His Word. You need to know the power of being in union with God, His Word, His work and His kids!

CHAPTER 6

Union With God, His Word,
His Work and His Kids

nion. Dictionaries have many definitions for the word *union*, but the very first one in the *American Heritage Dictionary* is this: "The act of uniting or the state of being united." The second is this: "A combination so formed, especially an alliance or confederation of people, parties, or political entities for mutual interest or benefit."[1]

Jesus was so connected to His Father, so united with Him in purpose and in thought that He said, "I don't do anything without my Father's approval; it's my Father in Me who does this work! All I am is a vessel for My Father to flow through." (John 14:10.) In John 10:30, He said, **I and my Father are one.**

You can't just believe this stuff. You've got to get beyond, "Oh, I believe it," into the realm of "I know it." Real belief isn't passive; it's active. *Knowing* something means that you've become involved. You've allowed it to become a part of you. You don't just believe it's true, but you know it's true!

When you *know* the power of God's salvation, you know that through the blood of Jesus the dominion of sin has left your innermost being. Yes, you can deliberately yield to sin, but it takes just that—a deliberate yielding. When a choice to sin is presented to you,

---

[1] *The American Heritage Dictionary of the English Language*, 3rd ed. (Boston: Houghton Mifflin, 1992), s.v. "union."

your spirit will quicken something in you and you will know what is the right choice. Your spirit knows what to do. Why? Because it is *united* to the very Spirit of God. It is *connected* to that Spirit. It is in *union* with that Spirit.

Real Unity

Unity is a fundamental basis of power within you and within the rest of the body of Christ. Now, you and I both know that Jesus said, **For where two or three are gathered together in my name, there am I in the midst of them** (Matthew 18:20). That's a powerful promise from God, and it shows us how important Christian relationships are to the Lord.

When we come together in the unity of Jesus' name, we create an atmosphere for God to move. We give Him an opportunity to be in our midst. This is why you see people healed so often when another person prays for them with the laying on of hands. There are two people uniting with the purpose of tapping into the healing power of the blood of Jesus. And that is a powerful thing to God. He recognizes unity, both in the physical presence of two people and in the spiritual presence of two people.

In other words, if you're fighting like cats and dogs with your wife and holding resentment in your heart for her, just because you say a nightly prayer together doesn't mean that you're coming together in the unity of Jesus' name. Your bodies may be there, but your hearts are far, far away from each other. And you're *not* in unity! The husband may be thinking, *Woman, you're nothing but a pain in my neck!* and the wife thinks the same thing! The Bible says that each spouse's prayers are hindered when the two aren't in agreement.

When it comes to the prayers of married people, 1 Peter 3:7-12 puts it in black and white:

> **Likewise, ye husbands, dwell with them according to knowledge, giving honour unto the wife, as unto the weaker vessel, and as being heirs together of the grace of life;** *that your prayers be not hindered.* **Finally, be ye all of one mind, having compassion one of another, love as brethren, be pitiful, be courteous: not rendering evil for evil, or railing for railing: but contrariwise blessing; knowing that ye are thereunto called, that ye should inherit a blessing.**
>
> **For he that will love life, and see good days, let him refrain his tongue from evil, and his lips that they speak no guile: let him eschew evil, and do good; let him seek peace, and ensue it.** *For the eyes of the Lord are over the righteous, and his ears are open unto their prayers: but the face of the Lord is against them that do evil.*

This Scripture is for married people, but what it all boils down to is forgiveness. Unforgiveness toward another person is a surefire way *not* to receive from God, regardless of your marital status. Just check out Mark 11:25-26:

> **And when ye stand praying, forgive, if ye have ought against any: that your Father also which is in heaven may forgive you your trespasses. But if ye do not forgive, neither will your Father which is in heaven forgive your trespasses.**

That goes for everybody, you know. Even the people you don't necessarily like. You don't have to like them. You don't have to hang around them every day. But you'd better forgive them if you want God to forgive you, because remember, without forgiveness you aren't righteous. And without righteousness, you don't have access to God. See the connection?

So check your heart. Go to God about it. Allow Him to help you get any hindering stuff out of your heart. That's called allowing Him to abide in that area of your life and wash it clean with His blood. There is no point in muddying up your prayers with stupid stuff like unforgiveness. Let God clean you out. Give Him every opportunity to open His ears to your prayers—forgive.

Unity of the Name of Jesus, Not Religion

I can hardly imagine what would happen if everybody who claimed Jesus was the Son of God came together in unity. Imagine the power of our prayers!

That would be a really hard thing to do today. It seems like people will gather together in the name of Baptist, Assemblies of God, Church of God, Word of Faith, Presbyterian, Episcopalian, Catholic and every other Christian religious sect. But few are putting aside their differing interpretations of God's Word and gathering together simply in the name of Jesus.

The Bible is an interpretive book. Until Jesus comes and sets us all straight, there is always going to be one group of people who interpret one Scripture to mean one thing and another group of people who interpret the same Scripture to mean something else.

A man asked me the other day, "Are you Word of Faith?" I could tell he was a little irritated about the prospect of my being in a group like that.

I said, "Well, what are you—Word of Doubt?"

I don't like to be labeled. I'm a believer. I love Jesus. Next question.

I believe that we're all Word of Faith! If you're a Baptist, it took the word of faith to be a Baptist. If you're a Methodist, it took the word of faith to be a Methodist. It takes the word of faith to be Catholic, Church of Christ, Assemblies of God or full gospel. It's *all* done by faith! So we're all word of faith. We all believe the Word by faith, so we must all be Word of Faith! What I'm saying is that I'm tired of people trying to separate the family. We are the family of God. Let's get together!

I realize that we may not be able to agree on a single religious affiliation. We may not all be able to agree on all the teachings of the Bible, but wouldn't it be nice if we could unite in our agreement that Jesus is Lord? Jesus is God's Son! Most Christian denominations agree on that—otherwise they wouldn't call themselves Christian. And isn't it enough for all of us to gather in His name?

I know some people who can't worship God with me. I've got a friend. I like him. He likes me. But when I asked Him to come and worship with me he was all shook up about it. He said, "Jesse, I just can't!"

"Why?" I asked.

"Because you believe in tongues. I think tongues are of the devil."

"Well, let me ask you something. Do you think I'm going to heaven?"

"Yeah, I know you're going to heaven."

"Well, if you can't fellowship with me here, how are you going to fellowship with me there?"

He blinked his eyes a little, trying to digest it. He was confused. I guess so—he was trying to understand a confusing doctrine. But regardless of whether he chose to believe in it or not, he could have come and worshipped with me.

Tongues—It's Not Just a Lot of Babbling

As for the issues of speaking in tongues, I can understand why people misunderstand. Really, it is sort of strange. Nobody can understand you, and it just sounds like a lot of babbling. But you know, I could say the same thing for the Chinese language. Or Russian. Or Italian. Or any other language that I don't personally know. You could too. If you're Spanish and you can't understand English, English just sounds like a bunch of babbling. If you're English and you can't understand Chinese, Chinese just sounds like a bunch of babbling. Do you understand what I'm trying to get across?

If you don't understand a language, does that mean it's a bunch of babbling? Does it mean that it comes from the devil? No. You just don't understand it.

I know that if tongues were of the devil I would have found them when I was living for the devil. I would have been the most tongue-talking man on the planet, because I served the devil with some serious gusto! I loved sin. It was my favorite thing to do.

I lived to get drunk, take drug trips and run around with women. I was crazy. I'd do anything. I used to love to take PCP, a hallucinogenic drug, and I thought it was hysterical to give it to unsuspecting people. At the clubs they used to have popcorn in these bins. I'd throw PCP in the popcorn bin. People would be crunching on popcorn, and suddenly they'd be high as a kite. I thought it was the funniest thing in the world. They'd fall off the barstools, and I'd just crack up.

I was a rock musician, and the girls just loved that. It was fine with me. I'd slide on over, drunk as a skunk, and say, "Whatz happnin, Mama?"

If tongues were out there, I would have found them.

But they weren't.

Tongues were just in the church.

Personally, I believe that tongues *are* for today. I don't believe that they passed away with the first set of Christians. I don't believe that the devil resurrected them and is passing them off in churches across the world. When was the last time the devil gave you something that actually drew you *closer* to God?

The act of speaking in tongues is what many call the evidence of the baptism of the Holy Spirit—the immersion in God's presence. Although the Holy Spirit immediately comes to live in every person who receives Jesus as Lord, something different happens when a person is immersed, or baptized, in God's Spirit. Really, people are trying to get closer to God, and somehow when they do reach out and completely yield to the power of His presence, these strange words kick in. And it does seem strange, but it is an amazing way to communicate with God.

I believe it is a way to communicate with God, because when we are seeking to do so, our language just goes bankrupt on us. There is no language anywhere on this earth that can express and hold the power of Jesus Christ. Tongues have got to flow out of you. They have to. All languages past, present and future cannot conceive or even begin to hold the greatness of God's power. It's that simple.

Now, you don't have to believe it. It's up to you what you believe. I can't force anything on you, and I don't want to. But even if you and I disagree with each other on this subject, isn't it possible for us to unite as believers? Sure it is.

Here's a little lesson for you, and it's important when it comes to your love walk. The next time your Christian friends or family members say something that you completely and totally disagree with, don't get all shook up and go into attack mode. Share what you believe. Do it in love. And if they don't accept it, don't keep homing in on them. Don't keep at them until they say, "OK, OK! Whatever! Leave me alone!" You'll just drive them away. But more importantly, you'll break down the union that you have with them in Christ.

Instead, say something like, "Well, at least we agree on one thing: Jesus is Lord, and He saves! Thank God for Jesus because hell sure is hot!" If you can, agree on something! If not, at least smile.

Sometimes it is good when people disagree with you. It stretches you a little. If anything, it makes you realize what you really believe, or else it makes you question and go searching in the Word. Either is good.

You are commanded to love—that's just the way it is. If you want God's presence in your own life, you've got to be in union with other people. Isn't it about time we all realized that? Isn't it about time we let our differences fall by the wayside and focused on what we do agree on—Jesus!

Unity With Jesus Obliterates Sin

When the Lord started speaking to me about unity, I said, "But I'm a flesh man." But then I looked at His Word and found out that He was too. Jesus left His rightful place in heaven and came as a flesh man to the earth. Yet He *didn't* sin.

The Bible says in Romans 3:23 that the rest of us have sinned: **For all have sinned, and come short of the glory of God.** All of us have messed up. None of us is perfect. But do you realize that as a born-again believer, you are so united with Jesus that if you talked about your past sins to God He wouldn't remember them? It is true! He has the power to blot things out of His memory and cause Himself to forget! He is God, and He can do that.

The Bible says that He washes sin away from you, never to be remembered against you anymore. (Hebrews 10:17; 1 John 1:7.) That sin is thrown into the "sea of forgetfulness." You can't be held accountable for it anymore. That is the mystery and greatness of the blood of Jesus! You've united with Christ Jesus, and His blood has washed you clean of all sin. Your unity with His work on the Cross obliterates all sin.

The Union of Jesus and the Father Is The Very Law of Life and Fruitfulness

You don't need to sweat it, because God does the work! God established the law of life and fruitfulness, and it's only through union with His Son that you can produce any fruit at all.

In John 14:10 Jesus said, **Believest thou not that I am in the Father, and the Father in me? the words that I speak unto you I speak not of myself: but the Father that dwelleth in me, he doeth the works.**

God did the work when Jesus was on earth. Every miracle performed and every healing that occurred at the hand of Jesus was done by the Father God. The Father God made it possible to break every natural law through the birth, life and death of Jesus.

The same will be true with you.

You're a vessel, or a container, for God. He is the amazing life substance that fills you. It is the miracle of life that animates your physical body and gives you life.

You could think of it this way. You're the car that is driving God around. He's taking a ride in you. When you let Him in and allow Him to take hold of the wheel, He'll take you places you've never been!

Where will He take you? To the place where natural law is broken. To the place where sickness can no longer stay in your body.

To the place where addiction can no longer control your life. To the place where you are abiding in Him and His words are abiding in you. The place where you can ask what you will and watch Him do it for you!

Are You One With Christ?
Then You Should Be One With His Work!

The writers of the New Testament often used the words *in Christ* to describe their dedication to Jesus. They recognized Him as the Christ, the anointed One. While others called the writers of the New Testament "Christians," they chose to say that they were "in Christ."

Being in Christ meant that they had dedicated their lives to the cause of Christ. Their lives revolved around Jesus. They spent their lives dedicated to telling others about Him and following His teachings personally. In other words, they were abiding in Him, and His words were abiding in them.

Those early Christians didn't become one with Jesus only by accepting salvation through His blood; they became one with His *work* too. They became one with *all* the work He did at the Cross— not just salvation.

What is the work of the Cross? Again, Isaiah 53:4-5 prophesied it:

Surely he hath borne our griefs, and carried our sorrows: yet we did esteem him stricken, smitten of God, and afflicted. But he was wounded for our transgressions, he was bruised for our iniquities: the chastisement of our peace was upon him; and with his stripes we are healed.

As for the early Christians, they sought to do what Jesus had done. They sought to say what He had said. Did they overstep their bounds by trying to act like Jesus? No! He told them to! They chose to believe the following words, knowing that they could do even greater works by the power of God: **Verily, verily, I say unto you, He that believeth on me, the works that I do shall he do also; and greater works than these shall he do; because I go unto my Father.**

You Can't Divorce Jesus From His Word or His Works

Do you want to be healed or delivered? Then you can't divorce Jesus from His Word or His works. You've got to be one with Jesus' Word *and* His works. You've got to decide that if you are a part of Christ as His child, then you must be a part of the work He has set out to do on the earth.

What were His works? Well, they were many. But the main ones He told us to do were those in Matthew 10:8, which says, **Heal the sick, cleanse the lepers, raise the dead, cast out devils: freely ye have received, freely give.**

What did Jesus do? He healed the sick, cleansed the diseased, raised the dead and cast out devils. What did Peter, James and John do? They healed the sick, cleansed the diseased, raised the dead and cast out devils. What did the apostle Paul do? He healed the sick, cleansed the diseased, raised the dead and cast out devils. What happened? They broke the power of natural law with their belief in the power of God!

When Jesus told us in John 14:12 that if we believed on Him we would be able to do *greater* works than even He did, He said it because He knew He was going on to heaven pretty soon. He had only three years of time to do good works on the earth and tell people the truth about God. Think about that. Only three little years, and today, almost 2000 years later, we are still talking about the works He did. If Jesus could do all that in just three years, what can you and I do in a lifetime?

If we weren't in Christ, if we were not a part of His work, then He would not have told us to do these things. If we couldn't do it, He wouldn't have said it.

You and I *can* do these things. Jesus said we could, and He is not a liar. So if our purpose in life is to do the works that Jesus did—and even greater works than those—then Jesus has to give us the power to produce those works. And how did He give that power to us? By telling us what to do: **If ye abide in me, and my words abide in you, ye shall ask what ye will, and it shall be done unto you** (John 15:7).

I believe in accepting the Word of God at face value. If Jesus said it, then it is true. That's the bottom line. So the power to heal the sick is available in Christ, the power to cleanse the body internally is available in Christ, the power to raise the dead is available in Christ, the power to cast out devils is available in Christ. As we have freely received from God, so we should freely give to others.

Jesus Didn't Sweat Doing the Work— Even Casting Out Devils!

How could people get healed so easily with Jesus? How could He break natural law so easily? Was it simply that He was the Son of God? Well, you'd think it would be. But the Scriptures tell us that He left His position to come to earth and become a man. He called Himself the Son of Man. *We* call Him the Son of God.

Jesus agreed with those who called Him the Son of God, but He chose to call Himself the Son of man. I believe He was proud of His status as a man. He enjoyed being one of us. He just took it to another level. He showed us how much was possible, even with sin running rampant in the earth.

How could Jesus say such phenomenal, powerful things so easily? They'd just roll off His tongue like nothing—like when He told us to do like Him and **raise the dead**! (Matthew 10:8.) Whoa—raise the dead! I have to admit, my faith isn't there yet. I've never raised the dead. It's beyond me now. But wait—a day will come when my faith will be there. One day, I'll break the power of *that* natural law!

What about when He told us to **cast out devils?** Now, *that* I've got faith for! I'm not afraid of a bunch of slimy, fallen angels who like to play games. I remember that when I first got saved, they freaked me out. I read Matthew 10:8, and I thought, *No, I don't want to mess with devils.* I thought about Dracula and Frankenstein and thought, *Uh, no, I believe I'll pass on that.*

I'll never forget the first time I saw a person who was demon possessed. I was a newborn baby Christian. I had my diapers on. I wasn't quite in union with the Lord. I was saved. That's all I knew.

I was in church, and suddenly this woman started writhing and talking with this demonic voice. The elders of the church latched on to that woman and were going to town casting the devil out of her!

I couldn't believe my eyes! I'd never seen a possessed person before, and the awe I felt came right out of my mouth in the form of a big, loud "Whooooaa!" I guess I said it pretty loudly, because I caught her attention. And do you know what happened next? That girl turned and looked me straight in the eyes! And in the most evil-sounding voice she said, "Whaaaat?"

I thought I had soiled my newborn baby Christian diapers!

I cried out, "Nothing! Nothing! Nothing! I'm going home. I'm going home!" and sure enough, I left! It scared me. It scared me so badly. I thought to myself, *A devil asked me "what?"*

Now that I've gotten more united with the Spirit that is in me, I don't run from demons. I don't run around looking for them, you understand. But I don't run from them if they happen to rear their ugly heads. They're not beyond my capacity to handle anymore. My inner character has changed a bit concerning them, and I don't run out the church doors paralyzed with fear.

God Knows the Inner Character of Every Person

God knows your inner character. He knows your personality. He knows right where you are mentally and spiritually. He knows what you can handle emotionally. In other words, God knows what you are capable of, and He won't ask for more than you can do. He may want you to stretch a bit, but it's all within your reach.

What has God asked you to do? He has asked you to draw closer to Him, to abide in His presence. Is that something you can do? Yes, it is. You were created to be in contact with God. You may be out of practice, or you may never have considered it at all; but it is still a vital need of your spirit, soul and body.

God loves you so much and wants to take you beyond intellectual acceptance of His Word. He wants to take you beyond what you've been taught about Him. He wants you to *know* Him, not just know *about* Him. In my last book, *God Is Not Enough, He's Too Much*, I dealt a lot with that. If you don't know God, then you'll have a hard time believing His Word. You'll be full of man's ideas instead of the truth. It's important that you know the inner character of the Lord. In other words, what is He *like?* You can only get that knowledge by spending time with God. That is the only way to get to know Him.

In the Garden of Eden, God walked with Adam in the cool of the day. (Genesis 3:8.) Together they had fellowship, a relationship that was intimate in that they spent time with one another.

I believe that spending time with God in prayer and just being aware of His presence during the normal day literally keeps you healthy. We're tender beings in that *without* the water of the Word, we dry up. Without the fertilizer of God's presence, we dry up.

Union with God is essential to our growth as people—not just spiritually but physically as well. The Scriptures confirm it in many places. Just read the well-known Psalm 91, and see how much abiding in God's presence can do:

> **He that dwelleth in the secret place of the most High**
> **shall abide under the shadow of the Almighty. I will say of**
> **the Lord, He is my refuge and my fortress: my God; in him**
> **will I trust. Surely he shall deliver thee from the snare of**

the fowler, and from the noisome pestilence. He shall cover thee with his feathers, and under his wings shalt thou trust: his truth shall be thy shield and buckler.

Thou shalt not be afraid for the terror by night; nor for the arrow that flieth by day; nor for the pestilence that walketh in darkness; nor for the destruction that wasteth at noonday. A thousand shall fall at thy side, and ten thousand at thy right hand; but it shall not come nigh thee. Only with thine eyes shalt thou behold and see the reward of the wicked.

Because thou hast made the Lord, which is my refuge, even the most High, thy habitation; There shall no evil befall thee, neither shall any plague come nigh thy dwelling. For he shall give his angels charge over thee, to keep thee in all thy ways. They shall bear thee up in their hands, lest thou dash thy foot against a stone. Thou shalt tread upon the lion and adder: the young lion and the dragon shalt thou trample under feet.

Because he hath set his love upon me, therefore will I deliver him: I will set him on high, because he hath known my name. He shall call upon me, and I will answer him: I will be with him in trouble; I will deliver him, and honour him. With long life will I satisfy him, and shew him my salvation.

Union with God is a fundamental basis of power within you. Unite yourself with God, His work and His kids, and you'll be tapping into His very ability to break the power of natural law!

Your Body: The Thermostat

God created you to live forever. That's why your body rejects death with all its got. It fights death. It doesn't like death one bit. Your body does everything it can *not* to die. It was created to rejuvenate itself and fight off sickness and disease. Why? Because God created you to live.

Your body was created to line up with the Word of God. It was created to obey *you*—and the truth is that the body works better when *you're* obeying God. Proverbs 23:7 wasn't put in the Bible for nothing. It says, **For as he thinketh in his heart, so is he.** That Scripture is as true as true can get. Your physical body reacts to what your mind is producing. Your brain is hooked up to the rest of you, so whatever you're thinking affects the rest of you. It sends signals out that tell your body what to do. God created it to do that.

Have you ever seen someone with a cast on a broken arm squirm when somebody says the word *itch?* They may not have been itching at all, but suddenly their mind takes hold of the word and creates an itching to scratch! Or when you were a kid, did you ever play sick to stay home from school and you worked so hard at acting the part that you actually started to feel sick? What if your boss comes in angry and says he wants to see you after lunch? Your mind starts working, and soon enough, you're sweating!

Your Body Is a Thermostat

Your body will listen to whatever your mind says and do its best to comply with what it is being told to do. It is like a thermostat hooked up to an air conditioner unit.

If you set the thermostat in your house to air-condition and put the lever on 68 degrees, that compressor in your backyard is going to work until your house is cooled to 68 degrees inside. I don't care if it's 104 degrees in your house when you flip the switch; the thermostat tells the compressor, "Cool this place to 68 degrees!"

If you were to go out and look at that compressor, you'd see it sweating and groaning and working like a dog! The thermostat rules the compressor. The compressor listens to the thermostat's gauge. That compressor will burn up before it stops trying to complete the task required of it. It will get to 68 degrees, or it will die! That's how it's built to operate.

You're the same way. God gave you a thermostat called faith. Your body is just like a compressor—designed to obey faith in God. Once you set your faith in line with the Word concerning healing and keep it there, your body will produce what you set your faith for. It has no other choice. It's how God made you.

Your mind has to tell your body to shape up! It has to line up with God's Word! But your mind can't think one thing while your mouth says another. Confession won't change a thing if you don't believe what you're saying. You have to agree with what you're saying for confession to work! Faith goes to work when your mind and your mouth agree with your spirit! Results come when *you* agree with *you!*

When you're in union with the Word and you're unwavering in faith, you're telling your body, "Listen here, body. The Word says you're healed, so start producing!" It's like a thermostat set for success! It's going to get to the place of health!

Wavering day to day only prolongs the manifestation of God's promise in your life. It could be compared to starting and stopping your thermostat all day long. If you keep messing with a thermostat, it will take forever to get to 68 degrees, and it may never get there. Or it may burn up trying from all the stops and starts. Do you understand?

What You Feed Your Mind Determines Your Thoughts

What you feed your mind determines what your body will do on the inside. That is why allowing God's Word to abide in you is so important. If you constantly think, *I'm so sick and tired,* or *I'm so fat and unhealthy,* or *I'll never get healed,* or *I'll never be off of drugs,* or *Nothing works for me,* or whatever, you're not giving your mind any good direction. It will respond physically to that stuff. You'll stay sick and tired, fat and unhealthy, addicted and depressed. You're not giving your mind anything to work with! How can you expect to get healed with that mess confusing your faith?

Most people will say what they think. They may fake faith some of the time, but if you hang around long enough, whatever is in their minds eventually comes out their mouths.

If your thoughts are filled with all that negativity and confusion, you're sending signals to your body. Then if you speak it out, you're confirming those thoughts by giving them the power of words. And don't think that words are not powerful, because they are. Consider Proverbs 18:21: **Death and life are in the power of the tongue: and they that love it shall eat the fruit thereof.**

There goes that word *fruit* again.

This Scripture basically says that if you speak death, you obviously love it and will get it. If you speak life, you obviously love life and will get it. Do you see how far your thoughts can carry you? Do you see how powerful words are?

Don't Lend Your Tongue to What You Don't Want

A lot of people seem to love sickness. They talk about it entirely too much. It is the focus of their lives. You can ask them, "How are you doing?" And they'll reply, "Oh, I'm OK I guess. You know my back is pretty bad, and it's been giving me a hard time lately. And did you hear about so-and-so? He just got out of the hospital..." It seems like they live to talk about sickness and death.

Proverbs 18:21 implies that if you give the power of your tongue over to a subject long enough, you are showing that you love it, and eventually you'll eat the fruit it produces.

Fill your mind with the living, breathing, active Word of God so that your mind has something to work with! Read and reread the stories of Jesus' healings. Quote Scriptures on healing and health to yourself until you know them. Put your mind on something that will pay off.

(At the end of this book I've listed a number of Scriptures that will help you. They're all in the *King James Version*, so you may want to check other versions to see which one you can apply best to your situation.)

Results Happen When Your Mind and Your Mouth Line Up With God's Word

You can say, "I'm believing," until you're blue in the face. But if your thoughts don't agree with your mouth, nothing is going to happen. If you don't really believe your own words, you're praying without a foundation and you're internally confused.

Your body listens to your mind and your mouth. Think good thoughts, and you'll talk good talk; and good will come to pass. The devil may fight you, but he won't be able to stop you! He only has the power to hinder you. Only you can give him the power to stop you. And you do that with the words of your mouth. Death and life are not in the power of Satan. They are in the power of *your* tongue. And your tongue will follow after your mind. If your mind is confused, your mouth won't agree with it.

You may know in your heart that all this is true, but you've got to renew your mind if you want your body to fall in line. That's what I'm talking about here—unity. When you unite with God, He touches that natural law with His supernatural power, and *wham!* the natural law breaks!

Suddenly, feeling comes back into your legs. Where there once was a feeling of nothing, a feeling of something takes over! I don't care if a spinal cord is damaged and the whole body is shut down. One touch of supernatural power can heal the spine and straighten every bent limb! I don't care if cancer is in the last stages and you're ninety pounds. One touch of supernatural power can obliterate the source of cancer and make every rebellious cell start working right.

Some people think that getting their healing is hard. Well, it may seen hard sometimes. But I believe that when it is hard it is usually that there is 1) a lack of knowledge or 2) a lack of faith or 3) an abundance of double-mindedness concerning God's ability or will to do what He said. Most of the time the problem is getting the heart to line up with the mind so that there can be a clear focus on God's Word.

Do I think it's hard? I think that sometimes it is hard to believe and get in union with God. The world talks so much trash that you start believing it. But is it hard to receive the healing? *No.* Once you get in union, it isn't hard to receive healing. That comes from the hand of God, and He doesn't make anything hard. He only asks that you believe.

God's Will *Is* His Never-Changing Word!

Believing is hard for some because not only do they have a hard time becoming childlike but they also have a terrible feeling of unworthiness. They wonder if maybe it is God's will that they be sick, diseased or addicted. They wonder if maybe He sent problems to "teach them something."

God is good. If you don't believe it, just ask Him. He'll tell you. This world is bad. Satan is a serial killer. He is merciless and cunning and will even try to blame sickness and disease, which he brought into the earth with his sin nature, on God. He has even got Christians proclaiming his lies. Satan will do whatever he can **to steal, and to kill, and to destroy** your life, but Jesus came that you might have *life...and have it more abundantly* (John 10:10).

If you want to know what God's will is for you, check His Word. His Word *is* His will. It will never be His will for you to be sick, addicted, poor or without hope. How do I know that? Because He won't go against His Word. And there are Scriptures that give you a way out of every one of those situations. He wouldn't have given you a way out if He didn't mean for you to use it. It's your job to search the Word and find out His will.

His will isn't some illusive, secret thing. It's been around for thousands of years. And He isn't changing: **Jesus Christ the same yesterday, and to day, and forever** (Hebrews 13:8). Jesus' will is the same today as it was way back then when He said those words.

John 1:1 says, **In the beginning was the Word, and the Word was with God, and the Word was God.**

The Word *is* God. He is one with His Word. He won't go against it.

So if you read that Jesus healed someone in the Bible, you can be assured that He is willing to administer His blood to heal you too. If He delivered someone in the Bible, He will deliver you. How do I know that? Acts 10:34: **Of a truth I perceive that God is no respecter of persons.**

If you want to see natural laws break for you, you must be *focused* on what you believe—not *confused* about what you believe.

God's Trinity Doesn't Argue

The members of the Holy Trinity never argue with one another. They are in unity. You never hear of God saying, "Now, Jesus, why are You always coming to Me with these prayers? Don't you know

I'm tired of handling everything? Can't You just do something by Yourself for once?"

You never hear of Jesus saying, "Why can't You go down there to earth and do it Yourself, Dad? Why am I the One who has to get crucified? What if I don't want to be the Mediator? Ever thought of that, Dad?"

You never hear of the Holy Ghost saying, "How come I never get to say anything? How come I'm always just 'there'? Why can't I *say* something? I want to let You both know, I'm the One fluttering over the waters here! How come God got to say, 'Light be!' You know how hard it was to keep up that creating thing? It was hard to get this earth flowing and moving. Do You know how hard it is to always be dealing with sinners? It isn't easy, You know!"

Sounds funny, huh? But do you realize that you do that with *your* trinity? You argue with your body. You argue with your spirit. You listen to your soul spew off whatever it feels when you ought to be listening to the re-created spirit within you. Oh, that's strong, I know, but stay with me on this one!

Your spirit is in 100-percent contact with the Lord. It will flow right up to meet God, given the chance. It is in perfect union with God, but your mind says, *Let's not get crazy with this thing. You know how God is. Sometimes He does listen, sometimes He doesn't. Do you feel like a fool today?*

I know some preachers who skirt away from the "hard cases." They'd rather just pray for the easy ones. You know, the ones that can't be proved—the inner healings. They think that if they pray for someone in a wheelchair and that person doesn't come out of it immediately, the prayer was amiss.

They're wrong.

The evidence does *not* have to be seen immediately; all it has to do is be spoken. If we don't see it, that doesn't mean it isn't happening. Think of a pregnant woman. She's pregnant the day of conception, but does her belly swell in an hour and a baby come flying out? No! Inner work happens first.

As humans, we work from the inside out. That's how God created us. Inner healing always takes place before the outer healing. For example, you eat less for awhile before that weight starts coming off. You decide to do something before you do it. Your mind tells your body what to do, and so on.

Healing can come immediately, and then it's called a miracle. It can come over the course of minutes, hours or days. I've seen people receive healing immediately, and I've seen people receive healing day by day, getting stronger and stronger. Yet regardless of the time frame, it takes the power to break natural law to receive healing from God.

God Created You To Be in Unity With Yourself

God created you to be in unity within your very self. We've established that the body is the follower. The spirit is the part of you that holds life. The spirit and the soul are so connected or intertwined that the Bible says the only thing that can divide them is the two-edged sword, the Word of God. (Hebrews 4:12.)

If you allow your soul to always be at odds with your spirit, then you're not in unity and your body will follow whichever is the strongest. When you're united, your spirit, soul and body are working together, and you are extremely strong. You can kick the devil's brains out from now until Sunday and still not be worn out! Why? Because you're united. And there is power in unity.

Have you ever heard the phrase "A house divided against itself can't stand"? Jesus said it more than once. (Matthew 12:25,26; Mark 3:24,25; Luke 11:17,18.) Jesus wasn't double minded. He knew what He believed and established His union with God by eating, breathing and sleeping faith in God and love for people. That kind of focus makes things happen. That kind of focus breaks the power of natural law.

Jesus is our greatest example of unity, focus and strength. I encourage you to make a commitment today to release all double mindedness. I encourage you to renew your mind with God's Word and unite it with your spirit so that your body, the thermostat, hooks up with God's will for your abundant life. See for yourself how extraordinarily peaceful it is to have an undivided heart. There is nothing in the world that can compare to being one with God and one with His work.

Righteousness Breaks the Power of Natural Law

Have you ever noticed, if you're married, that the longer you're married the more the two of you start to think the same thoughts? You can finish each other's sentences, you know each other so well. After a while, you start looking alike, which is scary. Once you've had kids you start to call each other Mama and Daddy. Good Lord, I never thought that would happen! But it did, and it has stuck, even though our daughter has been grown and out of the house for many years now. I still call Cathy "Mama." I know a lot of men who do the same thing.

The funny thing is that after a while, you don't have to say a word to each other to get your point across. A look can do it. A gesture. You're in union. You're growing in fellowship.

Jesus was in fellowship with His Father. He was so close to God that He could pick up the slightest inkling that His Father wanted to do something. Jesus established His union with His Father by constantly doing acts of faith and love. Everything Jesus did and said was His fruit in life, and it showed that He was united with God. He wasn't united with God in the manner of Abraham or Enoch—these two had amazing relationships with God. But Jesus was different. He didn't mess up—*ever*.

Did Jesus have problems? Oh, yes. He had some serious problems. Did He have to fight off sickness? Yes. Disease? Yes. Lust? Yes. Temptation? Yes. The devil? Yes. Legions of devils? Yes.

The Bible says that He was tempted in *all* points as we are. (Hebrews 4:15.) That means everything. Everything that you've been tempted to do, He was tempted to do. But He *didn't* do it. He sinned not!

Isn't that amazing? That's the kind of God you and I serve!

Even when He came as a man and walked the earth, He was *still* strong! Even with all the temptations this world has to hurl at a person, Jesus was *still* strong! He was still blameless and sinless and spent thirty-three years without doing *any* sin. And He went to the Cross that way just so that *you* could break the power of natural law. Jesus was strong and righteous in His life and on the Cross so that in your weakness, you could draw from His strength.

Jesus Is the Mystery and the Majesty of God Within Our Reach

The grace of God is always around us, but it is Jesus who gives us the power to change through His righteousness! It is Jesus who gives us the power to connect with God's healing power!

As a born-again, "in Christ" man, I am unified with Jehovah! Elohim! Yahweh! He is within my reach! Me, a Cajun boy from the bayous of South Louisiana—I have the ear of God! Isn't that a kick in the head? I am *in Christ*, but I am also unified with His work.

If sickness tries to attach itself to my body, it doesn't stand a chance. The devil may fight, but he can't win, because I've got God on my side! And so do you!

People always say, "Well, why does that happen when you're a Christian?" Well, if the devil came against Jesus, the Son of God, why do you think he'll stay away from you? The devil is real. He isn't a rabbit in some fairy tale like *Alice in Wonderland*. This isn't Wonderland that you're living in! This is a sin-filled earth run by a fallen angel who hates the One who made you. That's the bottom line.

Living in this day and time, you'd better believe in Jesus! According to our own scientists, we're destroying our earth. They say the air is polluted and the water is polluted. Even the food we get at the grocery store is covered with carcinogenic chemicals. They say that the fertilizers sprayed on our fruits and vegetables cause cancer in rats.

Scientists say our soil is depleted of minerals. Our food is depleted of vitamins. The ozone layer has big holes in it, and we're cutting down all the oxygen-producing trees. I turned on the news not long ago and heard that the great city of Venice in Italy is being eaten up because of the pollution. Statues that have been there hundreds and hundreds of years are being eaten up. So you can imagine what the pollution is doing to the flesh of people who live there or anywhere near there.

All I have to do to see a chemical plant is walk out the front door of my house. The thing isn't any more than five miles down the road. Do I know what they're pumping into my air? No. I really don't want to know, to tell you the truth. I'd rather just trust God.

But let me give you some wonderful, wonderful news. If you're born again, Jesus, the hope of glory, is living inside of you! If you're dwelling **in the secret place of the most High,** you're going to **abide under the shadow of the Almighty** (Psalm 91:1).

There is no murdering pollution in the shadow of God. Jesus, the mystery and the majesty of God made within your reach, will keep your body healed! I believe that regardless of whether the whole world is going to pot, you can be the only one *not* sick. You can break that natural law and live in health.

The Same Spirit

The Bible says that if the same Spirit who raised Jesus from the dead dwells in (or inhabits) you, it will quicken (make alive) your mortal body: **But if the Spirit of him that raised up Jesus from the dead dwell in you, he that raised up Christ from the dead shall also quicken your mortal bodies by his Spirit that dwelleth in you** (Romans 8:11).

So even with all this pollution around you, all this radioactivity, even with the ozone layer "melting" before our very eyes, God Almighty has a complete robe of righteousness around you. It's God's glory, and it comes from being in His presence. It's invisible to you, but it's visible to God, keeping your body the way it should be, keeping your soul the way it should be and keeping your spirit the way it should be! Glory to God! Are you excited yet?

Crying about why you get sick won't fix a thing. Taking authority over it will! Dwelling in the secret place of God and then wielding the power of the Almighty will! That's why Jesus came! He came so that we would have the power to receive what we need to have— life and it *more* abundantly. (John 10:10.)

The Righteous Can Tap Into the Power

In the Old Testament, you couldn't touch God. His glory was so pure and refining that it would destroy a human body in a millisecond. Why? Because of old slew foot, Lucifer. His sinful nature had replaced the original nature of man. Man knew only good before Lucifer came to town, before he bit from the fruit (there is that fruit thing again) of the Tree of the Knowledge of Good and Evil. After man disobeyed God and sided with Lucifer, he inherited a sinful nature that couldn't stand up to God's glory.

The wall came down. *Whoosh!* Man couldn't communicate with God unless he was righteous. Innocent animals began to be slaughtered to atone for sin. To atone means "to cover up." God's people made sacrifices for thousands of years before the ultimate sacrifice came along—Jesus, the sacrificial Lamb. Jesus came along and made the final sacrifice for sin. And His blood did more than cover up your sin; it washed your sin completely away and made you righteous. That powerful, sin-cleansing blood made a way for you and me to be able to stand before God without guilt, shame or condemnation.

Jesus gave His life so that we could get back into right-standing with God and tap into His supernatural power. Jesus came to show us God's mystery and His majesty so we could touch Him and be made whole. And, brother, when He walked on the earth, you didn't need to touch His body. If you had faith, you could just touch His clothes and be healed!

A Woman With an Issue of Blood

I'd venture to say that the story of the woman with the issue of blood has been told millions of times. It's so famous because it shows how just a speck of faith and determination gets the attention of the Lord. Here is the story from Mark 5:25-34:

> And a certain woman, which had an issue of blood twelve years, and had suffered many things of many physicians, and had spent all that she had, and was nothing bettered, but rather grew worse, when she had heard of Jesus, came in the press behind, and touched his garment. For she said, If I may touch but his clothes, I shall be whole. And straightway the fountain of her blood was dried up; and she felt in her body that she was healed of that plague.
>
> And Jesus, immediately knowing in himself that virtue had gone out of him, turned him about in the press, and said, Who touched my clothes? And his disciples said unto him, Thou seest the multitude thronging thee, and sayest thou, Who touched me? And he looked round about to see her that had done this thing. But the woman fearing and trembling, knowing what was done in her, came and fell down before him, and told him all the truth. And he said unto her, Daughter, thy faith hath made thee whole; go in peace, and be whole of thy plague.

Now, how could this happen? What happened that allowed this woman who'd spent everything she'd had on doctors and suffered for twelve long, bloody years to get healed? What made this woman draw on the power of virtue when throngs of people were pushing against the master?

Yes, she had faith. But she also had something else—determination. She was willing to claw her way through the crowd, even if that meant she had to put her face down to the dirt. This woman didn't care if the crowd looked down on her. She didn't care if she got trampled on her way to Jesus.

This woman was *serious* about her healing.

She had a "whatever it takes" mentality. Her mind was not confused with, *Is it the will of God?* Her mind wasn't weighted with, *I'm so sick, nothing will work for me.* She seized the moment and refused to allow depression about her circumstances to steal her opportunity. She had a clear, concise objective. She knew that if she could just touch but the hem of His garment, she'd be healed!

Consider all that. This wasn't a woman who went up to the altar to get prayed for but got mad because the preacher didn't talk to her. She wasn't a woman who got angry with the ushers. She didn't care if there was a 400-pound man slain in the Spirit beside her who smelled of garlic and sweat. Funny as that seems, there are a lot of people who desperately need healing who just aren't desperate enough for it. They're not focused on healing. They're focused on the external situation.

Now, this woman with the issue of blood wasn't a poor, downtrodden woman who'd never had anything in life. Obviously she'd had money at one time, because the Bible says she spent all she had over twelve years. Twelve years is a long time. This woman had spent all her money on doctors! And what good did it do her?

Well, I'd say that the woman with the issue of blood gave doctors some pretty hefty donations, and she did for over a decade. I guess you could say she was supporting the medical field and helping doctors to advance their scientific techniques. She was a guinea pig. And in the end, she came out just as sick as ever, but broke too. Sound familiar?

Be It According to *Your* Faith

God is the best specialist. He knows what's going on inside of you, because He made you! Now, I'm not against medicine. When people ask me that question, I just quote Matthew 9:29: **According to your faith be it unto you.** I believe that God will use medicine if you put your faith in Him to make the stuff work. After all, most of it came from plants God made, so I don't think He's against your using it if it will help. If you're having a problem receiving and there is medical help out there, do what you can in the natural until you get a revelation and can tap into the *super*natural.

My problem is with doctors who are *practicing* medicine. I don't want anybody practicing on me. I want doctors who know what they're doing! And if they're just practicing, how about a thirty-day guarantee? If you can't fix me up in thirty days or fewer, I want my money back!

Don't tell me, "Take this medicine. It's gonna cost you some, and we don't know if it's going to work or not. But if it doesn't, we'll try another one." Well, if it isn't working, give me my money back!

After paying through the nose, I at least expect them to know what they're doing! All that aside, I'd just rather go to Jesus. Jesus knows what He's doing! Jesus doesn't have to issue a guarantee! He isn't practicing medicine! And He doesn't charge an arm and a leg. It's free, but it didn't come cheap. It cost Jesus His life!

When that little woman came into contact with Jesus, the anointing of God in Jesus broke the power of natural law inside her body. *Wham!* The Bible says that the blood dried up that *same* day.

Figs Can't Heal Terminal Illness—Only God Can!

In 2 Kings 20:1-11 there is another story of breaking the power of natural law. This one has to do with figs!

King Hezekiah's time was up. He was sick and on his way to death when he fervently prayed to God about his situation. He poured his heart out to God, explaining how he had walked before the Lord **in truth and with a** [loyal] **heart** (v. 3). And God heard him.

It was Isaiah who told Hezekiah the news:

> **Thus saith the Lord, the God of David thy father, I have heard thy prayer, I have seen thy tears: behold, I will heal thee: on the third day thou shalt go up unto the house of the Lord. And I will add unto thy days fifteen years; and I will deliver thee and this city out of the hand of the king of Assyria; and I will defend this city for mine own sake, and for my servant David's sake.**
>
> 2 KINGS 20:5,6

Hezekiah sought the Lord, and the Lord heard him. He told God of his fruit in life, and God responded to it!

Another important thing about this passage is that after Isaiah delivered the word of the Lord, he used something as a medicinal agent, and Hezekiah was healed. He told Hezekiah to get a lump of figs and smear it on the boil. Now, some people believe that the figs healed Hezekiah, but I don't believe that.

While I believe the use of the figs was an act of obedience to the word of the Lord, I believe that it was God, not figs, who instituted the healing. Hezekiah might have put His faith in God to use the figs to help, but I don't think that figs themselves could have healed Hezekiah of a terminal illness! Hezekiah was flat dying! No fig, no matter how good, could change that fact! It could help him, but it couldn't heal him. Only God could change the fact that his time was up.

Don't misunderstand me though. I believe in medicine and the treatments we have available today. I think that many of them are wonderful ways to help heal our bodies. Medicines can help you greatly, and I believe God put things on this planet to help heal your body. But when a terminal illness has latched ahold of you, the only treatment you can really bank on is the Lord's.

But it is never good to fall into the trap of putting all your trust in a pill or a treatment. If you're terminally ill like Hezekiah was, God is the One who deserves your most trust. Put your faith in Him. Clean out your heart and show Him your fruit. He will answer your prayer! He may use a drug or a poultice of figs to help you out, but don't think for a minute that a medicine can do all the work— God is the One who orchestrates your healing. He is the One who breaks natural law! His will on earth is the same as His will in heaven—habitation!

Don't Let Your Circumstance Stop You!

Oh, the devil doesn't want you to hear *this!* That idiot is shaking in his horn-toed shoes, because when you get a revelation of who is inside of you, your faith is going to be ignited! You will be united in mind and spirit! And when you are, look out, body! That spark of faith is going to connect with the Most High, and you are *going* to break the power of natural law! *Suddenly* you will be made whole!

Getting Into Spiritual Shape

When I was in high school, I wanted to play football—bad. I didn't want to play for the game's sake. I could have cared less about winning. I was there for one reason and one reason only: girls.

Blood, Puss and Girls

Girls loved football players. I loved girls. I thought that was a winning combination, so I went out for the team. I got in. But not *really* in. I was small. But I had two things on my side—determination and enthusiasm. I was sixteen years old and ready for anything. The coach saw how determined I was, and I think that's why he took me in.

My uniform came in, and it was a beautiful, bright shade of white. I was so proud of it. I imagined in my mind how cool I was going to look after the game with my white uniform covered with mud and my hair all wet with sweat. Girls loved that. They loved to see a guy busting his can for the home team. I couldn't wait to run through the cheerleader section toward the lockers.

When I came for practice my coach handed me a dummy and told me to get out on the field. He told me that was my job for the day—to hold dummies for the players to practice hitting. "OK, Coach!" I hollered and ran out in the field with my dummy. *Wham!* They'd slam into me. I'd fall down, and coach would say, "Pick Jesse up!" I'd jump up on my own and say, "No, Coach, I'm up! Come on, send 'em at me again!"

I practiced playing with the team too. I'd run like fire down that field. I could run fast because I was little. But when I got tackled, it was pretty rough! My brain rattled, and my insides shook! These were some huge, monster-sized guys! They looked as if they ate guys like me for breakfast!

Game time came, and coach told me my position—the bench. If somebody got taken out of the game, I was in. Until then, I was to stay put. I really did want to play in the game, but it was obvious that I was the last choice, not because of my playing skills, because I wasn't bad. I was just too little. So I sat on the bench and watched, hoping for somebody to get knocked out.

The game was going on, and all the guys were really playing. They were sweating. The mud was dirtying up their uniforms. I sat on the bench with the whitest jersey ever made and looked over at the cheerleader section. They were rooting and hollering like mad-women. I looked at my gleaming white jersey. I looked back at them. Halftime was coming soon, and I'd have to run with the team back to the lockers.

I got an idea.

I rested my elbows on my knees and put my head down to contemplate it.

Yep. The mud was wet enough. Slowly I reached for the ground. Peering up to see if anybody was looking, I dug my hand into the mud and grabbed a big plug of it. As I pulled my hand up, I ran it up my leg. I looked down to see.

Hey, not too bad, I thought. I reached down for another plug. Then I took some of the water to drink. I raised it to my lips, and at the last second I threw it in my face. I ran my hands through my hair. *All right!* I thought.

Man, when halftime came the guys started running for the lockers, and I ran right along with them. I looked like I'd been beaten to pieces. The coach looked at me. I knew he knew, but those crazy cheerleaders didn't know.

I ran by them and got an intense look on my face. I let out a "Whew!" as if to say, *Man, I'm giving it all I've got!*

They started cheering, "Whooo! Keep it up! Make those touchdowns!"

"Yeah! OK! Thank you!" I said wearily as I jogged past.

When I got into the locker room coach said, "You get dirtier than anyone I've ever seen sitting on a bench." I just shrugged and said, "Yeah, I guess so."

I did that all season. And the cheerleaders never knew a thing about it.

One of the guys on the team was named Richard, and he was a 230-pound tackle. He was fifteen years old, but he was twice my size. I remember saying to him, "I wish I could play." He said, "I wish you could too, Jesse." Periodically throughout the season he'd ask me, "How come you get so dirty?"

I respected Richard. He was a nice guy and a great player.

Richard was big. He was heavy. I mean, he was so heavy that he couldn't run that much. Running wore him out, and he couldn't run laps like the rest of us. But if you had to try to run through him, that was it. You didn't go anywhere else. You stopped right there. It was like flinging yourself into a truck. You just had no chance.

I'll never forget one time when our coach built a plywood chute for practice. He said, "Duplantis, come here!"

I looked at that thing and went, "Oh, man! Oh, man!"

He said, "Richard!"

I went, "Oh no, he's gonna get Richard!"

He said, "Richard, I want you to get on offense. Duplantis, I want you on defense. I'm gonna stand over you like this. I'm gonna say 'hit,' and I want you to hit him!"

"Jesse," he said, "I want you to drive Richard into the ground. Stomp him, boy! Knock him to the ground! Can you do that?" It really wasn't a question, but I answered anyway.

"You've got to be kidding me! I can't even pop a pimple on his face, man! How am I going to knock this 230-pound guy out?" I asked. Mine *was* a question.

He didn't answer me.

He looked at Richard and said, "Richard, if you don't drive this boy into the ground, I'll run you till you vomit!" (If you're a guy my age, you probably remember when football was like that! It was as if they were training you for the military.)

Richard went pale. He couldn't run for long, and I could see in his eyes that vomiting on my behalf was not an option. He looked back at me and said, "Jesse, I'm gonna have to kill you."

Coach yelled, "I want to see some blood!"

I had an idea.

I frantically whispered, "I don't want you to kill me, Richard."

He looked at me and said, "Look, I can't run, man. I can't run like that. I'm gonna have to nail you."

I pleaded with him. "Look, you want to see some blood? Just go over me. You understand? Go over me! I'll make sure there's blood everywhere. Just do it!"

Coach hollered, "Set!"

I kept on. "Just do what I said, Richard. Listen to me. I'll let you cheat off me in class, but just don't hit me full force. Go over me. Fall on top of me. Don't hit me too hard!"

I heard coach's voice abruptly holler.

"Hit!"

Richard ran straight at me, and *whomp!* he knocked me back. He hadn't hit me full force, but it was still a hit. *Bam!* I fell to the ground, and as I was going I ripped my nails down my face and slashed pimples. Pus and blood were everywhere! Richard was falling down on me as I did it.

Man, you should have seen the blood and pus! I came out from under Richard growling with blood streaking down my face!

Coach said, "That's what I want to see!"

Richard and I looked at each other and said, "All right!" I had busted every pimple I could, saved Richard from running and saved myself from getting killed. The plan worked, and coach never knew a thing about it.

Now, how could I fool those cheerleaders? How could I fool that coach? (Don't worry, I'm still on the subject.) I could fool them because they did not know my character. They didn't understand my character. They weren't in union with me.

With the Lord, only a personal relationship can develop increased fitness for service. He knows the inner character of *every* person. He doesn't just know *about* you; He *knows* you. You can't pull anything over His eyes! You've got to apply His Word to make it work. In other words, you've got to do more than just get on Jesus' winning team. You've got to get in there and play if you want to experience all the good stuff in God's Word!

Christianity Is About More Than Just Being on the Team

Everybody knows that it takes exercise to become physically fit. The body requires training to perform well physically. If you want to run a marathon, you'll have to spend some time training so that when the race comes, you'll be able to run it—and finish it without passing out! Wouldn't you agree that it is easier to run a marathon after years of training than it is to get up one day and try to make it through 26.2 miles?

Healing can be compared to this as well. A lot of people neglect to think about their health when they are healthy. It isn't until they get sick that they start trying to get fit, spiritually and physically, in that area of their lives. This isn't the easiest way to do it. It can be like climbing uphill, but many people have done it. It can be done!

Sometimes when the devil comes to steal, kill or destroy people's lives with sickness, they get caught "with their pants down." They don't have confidence because they haven't been exercising, spiritually speaking. They haven't been doing their aerobics! They haven't been flexing their muscles when it comes to the Word.

They're saved. They belong to the Heavenly Club. They've got their membership and the manual that comes with it. They can bring friends over, drink soda, eat ice cream and watch others play the game. But they're flabby, not fit. They can't perform what they are designed to perform. They can't do what others in the club are doing. They couldn't walk in a race, much less run in one. Why? No training. Lots of reading and talking, but little application. They are in union with Jesus but not with His works.

You can be full of the Holy Ghost and never exercise your full abilities. You can be saved and hear healing preached all your life and never exercise the power of God for yourself. If you don't exercise by becoming united with Jesus and His works, when Satan strikes at you, you'll be paralyzed by the blow. Or you'll try to muster up the guts to run him out of town, but you won't make it three steps into the sprint. Do you understand what I'm getting at here?

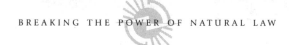

Be a Doer

James 1:23-26 puts it this way:

> For if any be a hearer of the word, and not a doer, he is like unto a man beholding his natural face in a glass: For he beholdeth himself, and goeth his way, and straightway forgetteth what manner of man he was. But whoso looketh into the perfect law of liberty, and continueth therein, he being not a forgetful hearer, but a doer of the work, this man shall be blessed in his deed. If any man among you seem to be religious, and bridleth not his tongue, but deceiveth his own heart, this man's religion is vain.

Religion won't do you any good unless you apply what it is teaching. You can read books like this one and hear a lot of soul-stirring sermons, but if you don't apply them, they can't work for you. That sounds like common sense—and it is—but a lot of people don't seem to understand how true it really is.

I know what it means to work hard at being physically fit. I've been a jogger since 1979. Have I enjoyed it? Not really.

My body is used to it. It doesn't like it, but it needs it—and it knows it. If I go for a couple of days without jogging, my body actually tells me, *Hey, fool, we're getting weak here.* Exercise helps me not blow up to 300 pounds, and it helps me to release stress. It's also a great time to talk with the Lord.

The first mile is not bad. The second mile is not *too* bad. But the third mile is a killer. My body decides it's had enough and says, *Hey, Jesse, look at your hair. It's white. You're getting old. You're gonna kill us out here on this road. What's the matter with you? Go home. Sit down.*

Eat. Who cares? I have to push myself to finish my course, because if it were up to my flesh, I'd be home in front of the TV eating pecans by the truckload and knocking the fire out of a bag of hog crackling. Oh, thank God for pigs!

Now, don't misunderstand me. I joke a lot, but I do try to take care of my body. When I don't, I just fall on the mercy of God, but I really do try to take care of what I can in the natural. Is it always fun? No, not really. Does my body like it? No.

Back when I was a strict vegetarian my body fought me tooth and nail. But it got used to the change. It got to the point that my body was so clean that if I ate just a bite or two of something fried I'd get an awful feeling in my stomach. I could taste the grease for hours, and it just wouldn't sit right in my body.

Sometimes I wonder if all that vegetarian stuff is nonsense. After all, look at my hair. Most people take one look at me and think I'm sixty years old. I've even had people at the movies give me the senior citizen's discount. I'm not a senior citizen—not at the time I'm writing this book anyway. I say, "Hey! I was born in 1949! Don't let the white hair fool you." They just smile and say, "Well, just go on. Don't worry about it." It bothered me at first, and then I thought, *What am I complaining about? I got in cheap!* I look at Cathy and say, "You should dye your hair white, woman. Save me some bucks!"

Cathy doesn't have one gray hair. Her whole family doesn't seem to get gray until they're past sixty. Me? I started getting it at thirty, and by the time thirty-five rolled around I was as silver as a fox. By forty-five, I was as white as Santa Claus. Now it's just getting more luminous by the year. I'm starting to glow. It must be the anointing!

Hey, don't smirk—Moses came off that mountain glowing. It could happen! But my point is that I'm in good spiritual shape! I've been abiding! How about you?

Lean, Mean Faith Machine

Getting in spiritual shape is a lot like getting in physical shape in that you feel wonderful when you're finally doing it! With physical fitness, your body moans and complains in the beginning. It doesn't want to do anything. But once you get into it, you feel good knowing that you're accomplishing something. You're gaining a healthier body, losing pounds and building strength and endurance so that you can enjoy your life more. You're being active. If you stick with it, it can transform your body into a lean, mean faith machine!

That's how it is with getting fit spiritually. At first your flesh moans and complains about making a change. It doesn't want to change. But once you get into the habit of crucifying that flesh, you feel wonderful because you are fellowshipping with the Creator! Suddenly He lifts you up into heavenly places, and it is no work at all! The difference between physical fitness and spiritual fitness is that getting fit with God is much, much more rewarding and fun.

Fight the Good Fight of Faith

Of course, being spiritually fit is not a complete safeguard against the devil's attacks. But when you're fit, it's a whole lot easier to whip him!

Satan is a stinking dirtbag. He's like a criminal who comes into your house to steal. He has no authority, but he'll try to get away with anything He can. It is our job to enforce the law of **by** [His] **stripes ye were healed** and kick the stinking sickness out. (1 Peter 2:24.) When we catch Satan trying to pull a shenanigan with our health, it's our job to grab the sword of the Spirit, the Word, with confidence and resist the temptation to give in. Sometimes it's a fight, but it is a good fight.

First Timothy 6:11-12 says,

> **But thou, O man of God, flee these things; and follow after righteousness, godliness, faith, love, patience, meekness. Fight the good fight of faith, lay hold on eternal life, whereunto thou art also called, and hast professed a good profession before many witnesses.**

There are some of those fruit of the Spirit again! And they are right there slapped up against **fight the good fight of faith!** That tells you something, doesn't it? Yeah, to me it screams one big word: Abide! When Satan comes to steal, kill and destroy, it's time to abide in Jesus and allow His Word to abide in you! That's how you win. You just keep abiding—whatever the circumstances say.

If you want to receive, you've got to learn to develop tenacity. Quitters can't win the fight of faith. They forfeit the prize when they quit. It's people who abide in God and have His Word abiding in them who are in good spiritual shape. They patiently fight the fight of faith and inherit the promise. Like Paul, they are the ones who end up calling it a *good fight!* Let's just face it, when you're in good spiritual shape, it's a whole lot easier to *fight good!*

God Loves You Enough To Heal You

Some people think God is so detached from us that He doesn't care about our sicknesses. That is not true. When Jesus was on the earth, He was in the business of healing. Wherever He preached, He healed. In fact, His first recorded sermon mentioned healing:

> The Spirit of the Lord is upon me, because he hath anointed me to preach the gospel to the poor; he hath sent me to heal the brokenhearted, to preach deliverance to the captives, and recovering of sight to the blind, to set at liberty them that are bruised, to preach the acceptable year of the Lord.
>
> LUKE 4:18,19

Jesus was anointed to preach! He was anointed to preach good news to the poor. (And what is good news to a poor man? "Ain't gonna be po' no mo'!") He was anointed to heal the brokenhearted. He was anointed to preach deliverance to captives. He was anointed to preach recovering of sight to the blind. He was anointed to give freedom to people who are bruised by life. He was anointed to preach the acceptable year of the Lord—which means the year when **the free favors of God profusely abound** (AMP). Glory!

Now, let's go back to John 15 and learn what it means to be purged! Yeah, you read right—we're about to start talking about the dreaded "v" word—*vomit.* We're going to learn how to get the urge—the urge to purge!

Getting the Urge—The Urge To Purge!

In Southern Louisiana, we eat something that a lot of people around the world grimace at the sight of. Crawfish. We love crawfish. We eat the tails and suck on the heads. Some of us suck the crawfish heads so hard we make their eyes click! Now, if you're not from here, don't start crinkling your nose just yet. You can't knock something until you've tried it.

If you haven't tasted crawfish from around Louisiana, then you are missing a little bit of heaven right here on earth. Think lobster but with more spice and a much more tender tail. Lobster is rubber compared to crawfish! I'd throw a lobster in the garbage can if I had to choose between the two. It's just that much better.

Of course, people from out of state rarely know how to prepare crawfish. I think it is a sin to boil crawfish anywhere but in Southern Louisiana, because others just don't have the talent for it! I'm just being honest here.

You wouldn't expect a person from the backwoods of Alabama to crank out a delicious meal of sweet and sour short ribs, hot and sour soup with tofu, egg foo young and shrimp fried rice, would you?

And you wouldn't ask a person from China to cook a Southern buffet of chicken-fried steak with white cream gravy, mashed potatoes, buttered field peas, homemade buttermilk biscuits and sweet potato pie, would you? Every group of people has their specialty—cuisine that only they do best. And here in Southern Louisiana, it is no different.

We do boiled seafood better than anyone, and we can cook up a chicken and andouille gumbo, crawfish bisque, crabmeat au gratin and fried oyster po'boy that will make you want to "slap your grandma," it's so good! I'll tell you what, a spiced-just-right boiled crawfish never tasted so good as here in Southern Louisiana!

But there are a few things you need to do before you can crack open the first tail.

What It Means To Really Purge

Around here, crawfish live in the muddy freshwater bayous. So the first thing you have to do is clean them up. Nobody just boils them outright. We don't eat what we call "dirty" crawfish. Before we eat them they must go through an external *and* internal cleansing. There is a process that must be completed before they are ready for the boiling pot.

First, you start with a big, deep, stainless steel round tub and fill it with clean water. Then you put the live crawfish in water. They just swim around and crawl all over each other. They don't know that hellfire is coming.

Then once they're completely submerged in the water, we start adding boxes of salt to the tub. We pour entire boxes of salt into the water with the crawfish. Now, these are freshwater crawfish. They don't live in salt water. And they can't take it. They start drinking in that salt water, and then they do just what you'd do if somebody made you drink a gallon of salt water. They start to vomit.

They go, "Whoa, man! What the heck is this?" The salt is like a drug to them. It makes them lethargic and slow because, basically, it's making them sick. Salt is a healing agent. It has a drying and cleansing effect to their systems. Whatever was recently digested will come out of those crawfish once they start sucking back that salt water. They vomit, and they vomit hard. We call it purging.

The salt water also gets into their entire systems, which not only cleans them out but seasons them too. Cajuns aren't stupid! We like flavor! Then once the crawfish have been purged, we take them out of the water and rinse them with fresh, clean water. It is only after the purging that we put them in a boiling pot, filled with more spices, onions, whole cloves of garlic, corn, potatoes and sausage. They're alive when they go in, and they're cooked to perfection when they come out! They're tender, spicy—a feast laid out on the table for everyone to enjoy.

Now, I know what you're thinking—*Cajuns will eat anything.* Yeah, you're probably right. But at least we clean our food inside and out before we eat it! Nobody has recalled crawfish from the grocery store yet! I haven't heard of anybody's keeling over from contaminated crawfish. Why? Because we kill everything inside them with good, old purging salt! That's why crawfish taste so much better here in Southern Louisiana. They don't have that grainy texture you find in other places like, uh—Texas! We clean them. We get all the impurities out.

Give Up Your "But..." and Purge Yourself of Past Fruit!

I believe that in John 15:1-3 Jesus equated purging a branch with being fruitful because He knew that in order to receive more, you'd have to give more. In order to produce more fruit, you'd have to be willing to give more fruit. Again, He said,

> I am the true vine, and my Father is the husbandman. Every branch in me that beareth not fruit, he taketh away: *and every branch that beareth fruit, he purgeth it, that it may bring forth more fruit. Now ye are clean through the word which I have spoken unto you.*

The fruit of our lives must continue to be brought forth, season after season in our lives. There is no such thing as holding on to past fruit. Once fruit is brought forth and ripened, it is taken away. We don't own the fruit of our lives. If people come to the knowledge of Jesus through our witness, they do not belong to us, even though they are our fruit. They may remain attached to us for awhile, but eventually they are taken away by God in order that they may become branches from the true vine, Jesus Christ. They become one with us as branches. And even though they are newborn Christians, Jesus puts them on an equal level with us. They go on to produce fruit of their own.

This is God's system. It is not right to attempt to hoard or hold on to our fruit, but it is our duty to give forth our fruit freely throughout our lives. If you find yourself saying, "I would give that up, *but...*" or "I would give them up, *but...*" you're just making excuses for why you don't want to be purged. But allowing God to purge you is the only way to move forward with Him in your life.

Life isn't about standing still; it is about moving forward. With God you really are either moving ahead or falling behind. If you want to move ahead with God in your life and receive His best, you've got to give up your "but..."! You must allow God to purge you of past fruit—whatever or whoever that may be!

Yesterday's fruit isn't the focus anymore. Today and tomorrow are what's important. In Philippians 3:13-14, Paul the apostle puts it this way:

> Brethren, I count not myself to have apprehended: but this one thing I do, *forgetting those things which are behind, and reaching forth unto those things which are before, I press toward the mark for the prize of the high calling of God in Christ Jesus.*

Stop the *Rot*—Purge Yourself of Impurity!

If we try to hold on to past fruit, it can only be destructive. Have you ever seen a piece of fruit rotting on the vine? This is what happens when we try to hold on to our fruit. We must allow the Lord to take care of it.

This is a great lesson for pastors and leaders, but it is also a great lesson for any Christian, any parent or any person who has contact with other people. We can't exercise control over anyone, because, frankly, it's not our job to do it—even if we want to! So this is what He means when He says He will take away our fruit as we produce it. We have to let go of our past fruit and allow it to move from being our fruit to being our fellow branch, equal in every way. This is God's plan, and we have to allow Him to do it so that we can produce more.

Not only is trying to hold on to past fruit destructive in the lives of others, but it is destructive in our lives as well. Why? Because you can't do it and win by trying to fight what God intended. It just doesn't work. It only makes you weak. It only causes you to wither and rot and fade away.

Stop the rot! Rotting begins when you don't allow God to do His work in your life. When you try to get around His plan, you stagnate and stop growing. You create an impurity in yourself, and you begin to bear bad fruit, or the works of the flesh, instead of the good fruit of the Spirit.

What takes care of impurity? You got it! Purging! As a believer, you just can't bear much good fruit if you are withering inside with impurities. You may produce a little, but those impurities hold you back from reaching your full potential. Those impurities steal your peace too. And on top of that, they hinder you from going full force for God.

Purging gets rid of the impurities of the works of the flesh so that clean, effective power is not stopped as it is coming into your life. Yes, you can stop the flow of God's power in your life by refusing to open up to God or to change your ways. Refusing to move ahead with God—by releasing good fruit and purging bad fruit—literally breaks the flow of God's power in your life. And it is His power that leads to your breaking natural law and receiving healing or deliverance, prosperity or salvation.

I encourage you to search your heart about this, and make a commitment to yield to His plan of purging out what is bad. It is the only way to receive what is good.

It Is Never Your Job To Purge Others

What I've found is that most people don't want to purge themselves; they just want to purge others. They're always trying to find the speck in their brother's eye, instead of concentrating on the tree stump stuck in theirs! (Matthew 7:3.) There is a fine line between trying to help people and trying to run their lives. You know the line because you know your own motives. But others may not. So it's a good idea to keep your nose out of other people's business and refrain from trying to control their situations.

You don't have to run people's lives for them. You don't have to be their mama or their daddy. You can give them words of wisdom and guidance and help them out in whatever way the Lord puts on your heart, but be cautious about becoming overly involved. Be wise. Make sure your motives are pure, and don't try to purge others. That's God's job. And that can be bad news not only for you, but for them as well. They may unconsciously make you their source, and you could be creating a person who is more dependent on a person than on God.

Watch out for the urge to purge others. Speak the truth, but let God do the purging. Only God can purge the right way anyway.

Darkness Can't Work in Light, But Light Can Work in Darkness

Have you ever noticed that light can work in darkness, but darkness cannot work in light? Have you ever had the opportunity to travel down into a cave? There are caverns and salt mines in the

United States that go deep into the earth. Even though you can be taken a 1000 feet into the darkness of the earth, if you're wearing a hat with a light you can turn the light on even in the darkest pit of the earth and see a shining beam of light. The light looks before you. But notice, the darkness can't really operate in the light, because the minute light is present, darkness leaves.

You can experiment with this for yourself. At night, go into the darkest room in your house and turn out all the lights. Watch the darkness rush into the room. Sit still, and see what it is like to be in the dark for a little while. Then throw on the lights. *Wham!* Light will fill up that place in a second! There will not be darkness in that room. Why? Because darkness must leave in the presence of light. Light can work in darkness, but darkness can't work in light.

Think about it. Have you ever heard of a flashdark? No! But you've heard of a flashlight, haven't you? That's because the principle of darkness overpowering the presence of light doesn't work. Only light can beam through the darkness; darkness can't "beam" through the light.

This means Jesus *can* work through vessels that are not completely pure. He can still work in vessels that are riddled with dark crevices of guilt or fear or even sin. There have been preachers who have fallen into sexual and financial sin. Can people get saved or healed in their ministries even though they had problems in their lives? Yes, because Jesus can work in vessels that are not completely pure. Of course, I'm sure He'd like to work in cleaner places, but He will work with what He's got. He will use whoever is willing to be used. That's not how I'd do it if I were God, but hey, who am I to question Him? He is God, and He can use whomever He pleases!

A minister friend of mine has a grandson who is a really cute kid. He has a statement that he makes when he is getting sleepy and needs a nap. He says, "Paw-Paw, dark's getting in my eyes." Now, that's a great definition of being sleepy, don't you think?

If "dark" is getting in your eyes, it's time to turn on the light of God. If darkness is cluttering up your mind, it's time to turn on the light of God's Word. That Bible is like a clean, hot beam of light, penetrating the darkness. It is like a purifying light that has the power to obliterate sin, sickness and disease and fill you with righteousness, health and joy.

Throw Up and Throw Out
What Shouldn't Be in Your Life

Only God and you can tell what is inside your heart. Only you two can know what is really going on in your life. Pastors, preachers, friends and family don't really know your heart. Only God does. And only you can allow Him to purge you of what doesn't belong in your life. You know what impurities you have. The Holy Spirit is the One who convicts the heart of impurity, and if you stop for a moment, that thought will immediately pop up in your mind. If you're honest with yourself and try not to explain it away, you'll know immediately what you feel conviction about.

When you go to God about those things and allow Him to reach into your heart and purge you of the root of those impurities, you'll feel the cleanness of God's purifying. You'll probably also cry a bit. If so, don't worry. It's normal!

Sometimes we feel remorse over our impurities. Sometimes we don't want to let them go, so we cry. Sometimes we feel bad for having them in the first place, so we cry.

There is nothing wrong with crying, even if you're a man, because what are tears but salt water designed by God to purify the eye? Think of that! Producing tears is an action that the body does when it wants to release raw emotion. It purifies your eyes and allows whatever is on your heart to move from the inside to the outside. It purges you.

After crying, how do you feel? Cleaner. Like you've emptied yourself of some of the raw emotion. You feel better. Well, that's just the physical part. When you truly release the impurities to God, He goes further and digs into your soul to scrub it clean. And nothing feels as clean as being flushed of impurities by your heavenly Father.

Have you ever heard people say they felt like a burden was lifted from their shoulders after encountering God this way? You can bet that what was really happening was something called purging. God was purging them of impurities and of all the miserable emotions that came along with them!

Don't be afraid to go to God with your impurities. Don't be afraid to confront what shouldn't be in your life. You can't move forward unless you get out the junk. That's just a fact. Once you decide to stop the rot, you'll be free and clean, able to move forward in your life, break the power of natural law and receive from God once again.

Every Time You Go to Church, You'll See Something in Your Life That Needs Tending To

I'm a believer in attending church. There is nothing like a group of people who are totally dedicated to God's work coming together under the roof of a building! There is power in that kind of unity, and I believe you should always attend services that are held in your church. If you're tuned in to what is going on, I can assure you that each and every time you attend church, you will find something in your life that needs fixing. Don't get under condemnation about it. Fix it!

It really is pretty simple. As things come up in your life, as you notice things that need fixing, fix them! As a Christian, you're growing in the maturity and stature of God, so you're going to find impurities in your life. It's essential to your progress to recognize those impurities and purge yourself of them as they come up.

Progress Isn't Possible in a Person Who Doesn't Recognize Impurities

A lot of people refuse to check themselves out for impurities. I call the stuff that keeps making them stumble *defects*. They need the restoring hand of God. I examine myself for defects on a regular basis. If I don't, they can creep up and mess up what I'm trying to do for God. So I say, "Lord, open the closets that I haven't seen inside of me, because if there are skeletons in there, I want to know about them so that I can get them out."

When we become introspective and examine ourselves, we give God the opportunity to help us grow. Personal growth can happen literally on a daily basis if you take time to examine your heart and your motives in situations. Although there are times in your life that you will feel dedicated to growing at a fast rate, for the most part you should exercise a little introspection every day.

I know for some people that is hard because they don't want to think about what is really going on. But if you need something from God, I suggest you do it. Regardless of what they say, ignorance is not bliss. It's just plain stupid.

There is nothing more stupid than choosing to be in denial to the truth. You can't rightly complain about your situation if you're not willing to do something about it. You have to face something if you want to change it.

If you're sick today and want to be healed, you've got to face the fact that the devil is attacking your body. You've got to face the fact that there is more to getting healed than just being saved. You've got to face the fact that faith matters. You've got to face the fact that forgiveness matters. You've got to face the fact that fruit matters. You have to face the fact that what you do really does matter.

Denial is a trap Satan uses to keep you from the truth. And it is an easy trap to fall into because, let's face it, who wants to look at his own faults? Who wants to change? The flesh wants to stay the same and harbor resentment toward this or that one and explain away why this doesn't work and that doesn't work, but when it comes down to it, the truth is that denial limits progress. Denial stifles success. You can't win a battle if you never face it. If you don't recognize the defects or the impurities or you live in a state of denial, you'll never come to that point where God can really work within you to the fullest extent.

Jesus Covered It All—All You Have To Do Is Believe and Receive

Jesus covered it all. Jesus redeemed you so that you could be clean. Asking for forgiveness is a part of purging. So why be weighted down with impurities when His blood is available to wash you clean spirit, mind and body? "Well, how do I get that?" you might say. Release! Purge!

For you to break the power of natural law in your body, you're going to have to be purged from unbelief. Unbelief has a seat in every church in America, a seat in every church in the world. Wherever there is faith, there is unbelief. It is the opposite of faith in God. It is doubt in God.

The devil will throw doubt in your mind and try to get you to believe His side of the story. The Lord doesn't force you to believe His side. He simply asks you to believe Him. He wants you to choose Him because you want to, not because He is coaxing you into it. Faith is a simple decision to believe His Word.

Some people say, "Well, did Jesus really mean what He said?" Of course He meant what He said! Jesus wasn't talking just to hear Himself talk. He wasn't just shooting the breeze and asking the disciples to record it. His Words were life lessons, the keys to receiving from God.

One of My Big Stumbling Blocks—Traffic!

All of us need purging. You do. I do. The greatest ministers and the holiest people in the world do. No one is without blemish. But we're working on it! That is our common thread.

As a Cajun, I know firsthand what it means to have a bad temper. Most Cajuns blame their tempers on their heritage. I did too, until God corrected me. I remember one instance when my daughter was a little girl. That was my turning point—my purging point, so to speak. It was the first time I noticed that what I really needed was a good, old vomiting session.

Now, I used to drive like a speed demon. If the sign said 55 miles per hour, I thought that meant 75 miles per hour. I was always on my way somewhere in a hurry. If I needed to get ahead in traffic, I'd yell, "Break check!" out of my window as I sped past the guy next to me and cut over into his lane. If people made me mad, which they inevitably did, I'd holler at them from inside my car. I'd have whole conversations with people who never heard a word.

One day I was on my way to the airport. I was driving, Cathy was in the passenger seat and my daughter, who was only seven or eight at the time, was sitting in the back seat. I was running a little late and ended up behind a grandma going way too slowly for a two-way, two-lane country road. The speed limit was 55 miles per hour; she was putting along somewhere in the neighborhood of 35 miles per hour. Now, I don't know if she was counting the blades of grass on the side of the road or reading all the signs along the way, but what I do know is that I was in a hurry and she was in my way.

I started mumbling out loud. I started twitching in my seat and swallowing hard. I was already late. What I didn't need was to miss my flight on account of some old bird on a Sunday drive.

I veered right.

She veered right too.

I veered left.

She veered left too. I was trying to pass her, but Grandma didn't care. Grandma was taking the road. Grandma was weaving where she wanted, swaying to her radio for all I knew. I clenched my teeth and barked, "What's the matter with you!" Cathy looked at me, pursed her lips and kept quiet. Jodi was fumbling with something in the back seat. She didn't seem to be paying attention.

I tried to pass Grandma again. No such luck. She swayed, taking just enough time to make me lose the opening to pass on the two-way road. The car in the other lane flew past us. I was stuck. It was clear. I couldn't take it anymore. I lost my cool.

"This woman's gonna make me miss this airplane!" I exploded, as I jerked up in my seat and clenched my wheel with both hands. I sat up close to the wheel and started to talk to Grandma.

"Get out the way, you old woman! You old bag! Get out the way!" I was hurling angry looks at her and moving from side to side behind her on the road. Cathy was tense. She looked out the side window, trying to ignore me. Jodi's eyes got as big as saucers, and she sat up to watch the show.

Of course, Grandma couldn't hear me. Grandma didn't even seem to notice that anything was going on at all. She seemed to be completely oblivious to the fury behind her.

"What's the matter with you?" I barked again. "They ought to take your driver's license away from you! That's what they ought to do with you! They ought to give you a bicycle and let you drive around an old folk's home! GET OFF THE ROAD!" I had completely lost it. I was hurling insults at that old woman and beating on my steering wheel like an idiot. I was in complete fury—when *it* happened.

Suddenly, Grandma lost her muffler. It just fell right off her gigantic Grandma car.

Clang! Clang! Clang! It hit the road. I tried to swerve to miss it, but *whap!* I rolled over her muffler. *Whap!* Not just one tire, but both tires—cut!

Two flat tires! I knew it! I could hear the rubber rip. Oh, I got mad! Not mad like irritated or angry. I'm talking snarling, rabid, boiling vexation. I can't really describe how I felt just then, except to say that a touch of insanity rose up in my heart. Seething with it, I screamed at her as my car skidded to the side, "I tell you what, woman! If I could catch you, I'd..."

"Tell her that Jesus loves her, huh, Daddy?" My daughter interrupted me and finished my sentence.

The words stopped me cold.

I looked at Jodi. I didn't say a word. I couldn't, really. I had a ball of anger and tension the size of North Dakota stuck in my throat, and my heart was beating 100 miles an hour. It was as if time stood still and the fury stood by, waiting to see what would happen as I bit my lip and teetered on the slippery edge of insanity.

Cathy looked at me. I could read the words scrawled on her face—*If it weren't for me, you'd be in hell now.*

God was purging me. And He used eight small words from a child to make me see it.

Nobody said a word as we drove to the gas station to get the tires fixed. Patience was being worked in my life. When I finally did get to the meeting, the Lord started to deal with me.

Jesse, He said, *we need to deal with this temper.*

"Lord, I'll never do it again."

Don't lie to me, Jesse. Let's get serious here. You need to get rid of this. People are noticing things. You are an example to your daughter.

"She won't remember it."

Yes, she will. Kids remember these kinds of things.

I thought to myself, *Yeah, You're right. Promise them a cookie, and if you don't give it to them they'll come to your door thirty-seven years later saying, "What about that cookie you promised me in 1974 at 8:30 at night?"*

Now, how do we get these impurities out of us? Purging. We've got to allow God to get into our hearts and find the root. What makes a man so angry and high-strung that he wants to murder an old lady just for driving slowly? Sure, it's normal to get aggravated. But rage is something altogether different. I was beyond just "having a temper"; that temper was controlling me and stopping the power of God in my life.

The tendency toward rage was something I needed to be purged of. It was an impurity, or a defect, which I needed to allow God to remove from my heart. That impurity developed over the course of many years. I had practiced having no restraint. And it started in my childhood, when I was just a little boy.

Purging Gets Rid of All the Impurities in You So That Clean, Effective Power Is Not Stopped

When you allow the Lord to purge you of impurities, you are making the way for more fruit to come forth in your life. The day you got saved was the day you were delivered. The day you got saved was the day you received healing. Just as a baby is born with all its parts, God gave you every tool you need to take care of your spirit, soul and body. That is the miracle of the work of the Cross.

The minute a baby is born, it has muscles, tendons and organs. It has little legs and perfect little fingernails. The baby has all the tools necessary to walk and talk, but it can't do those things just yet. Why? Because it needs nourishment. The baby needs strength. It needs to learn how to use those muscles.

That baby needs nourishment to become strong so that it can finish developing. One day soon, though, that baby will start crawling. And suddenly, you've got to take all your stuff out of your cabinets so the kid won't drink the washing powder and toilet bowl cleaner! They're curious!

The problem is that although they have all the tools to crawl and chew and eat stuff, they don't realize yet what is good to put in their mouths and what isn't. Dishwashing liquid is attractive to a toddler! So is bleach! Those bright-colored bottles under the kitchen sink are attractive to babies—that is, until they digest the contents and start feeling what they do to their insides.

The World Has Many Attractions, But It Also Has Many Dangers

Some things in the world seem as innocent to Christians as a colored bottle of detergent does to a baby. The world has many attractions like that. But they're also dangerous because there is an underlying current swaying beneath the surface of those attractions that can slowly wean you from godliness.

Satan is so sly. He's like a bug, hiding in the dark, waiting to come out and sneak around your house when you're not looking. Every once in a while he will get on your face while you're sleeping, but usually he is in the corner and only comes out at night. He knows that he will get squished if he shows himself in broad daylight.

That reminds me of something I learned in childhood. When I was five years old my daddy taught me to play the guitar. From that moment on, I spent a lot of time in my room playing, scratching my guitar against the walls and the furniture, just to hear the different sounds I could make. I enjoyed playing.

A lot of times I'd go outside with my guitar. I'd play, and people would give me a quarter or sometimes a couple of bucks. Consequently, I always had money even though we were dirt poor. When I saw how easy it was to earn money playing guitar, I started to look for other ways to make extra spending money. I was sort of an elementary entrepreneur. I'd do anything to make a buck.

In fact, one time my brother wasn't home, and I went through his closet. I gathered everything he had, went outside and sold it all within two hours. I had my own garage sale—but with my brother's stuff! My mama was furious, and I took the beating. But it was worth it because, after all, I was rich!

When I was in the third grade, I came up with an even better scheme to get more spending money. I started to see my big brother, Wayne, as a possible moneymaker. Now, Wayne was two years older than I was, and he could throw a punch better than anybody I'd ever seen. He was a fighting machine, and nobody messed with him if he didn't want to get hurt—and hurt bad. My brother could whip anybody. Not only was he good at it, but he liked it! That alone made him tougher. I think that sometimes he knocked kids out just for fun. Me? I didn't want to fight. I wanted to have fun and make money. It was a good thing because I was too little to ever be really good at fighting.

So one day a kid in school hit me, and I ran to tell my brother about it.

"Wayne, that kid over there hit me!"

"What? Where?"

I pointed, and Wayne hit. *Whack!* right across the chops! It was great. After that incident I started thinking, *Hmmm. This could work for other people. Wayne never asks any questions. He doesn't sweat the details. He likes to fight. And I need some money. I know people who could*

use a brother like Wayne. This school yard is tough, and they need protec-
tion like I've got. They need it so bad I'll bet they'd even pay for it!

And that's how it began. I told all my friends, "If you have any
trouble with anybody, and I mean anybody in this school, come
and tell me about it. I'll take care of your fights. Any problem at all.
Don't try to fight on your own. Just come talk to me, and I'll get you
some protection. It'll cost you a quarter." It wasn't long before I had
about $3.50 a week coming in! That was what you called high
rolling for a third grader!

So when one of my friends was being threatened, he'd pay up
his quarter and I'd run to Wayne.

"Wayne, that kid hit me!"

"Oh yeah? Where?"

"There! That kid in the red shirt!"

Whap! Whap! Whap! Wayne would knock his lights out! Then,
he'd ask me if I was OK. I'd say, "Yeah," and he would walk back to
his side of the school yard. That was that. I'd collect my money and
go on about my business.

Wayne would always ask me, "How come you always got
money, Jesse? How do you get it?"

"I dunno. All kinda ways. You want fifty cents?"

Now, what was happening with me? How could a third grader
figure out how to make money off fighting? Movies. I was super
impressionable, and I loved watching *The Untouchables* on television.
I kind of liked the way Al Capone looked. He had a better-looking

suit than Elliot Ness'. The gangsters had big, nice, shiny cars. They always had pretty ladies around them and wore nice suits.

I'd go to Sunday school, and my teacher would tell me, "You know, the Bible says you should bless your enemies. Don't you want to do that, Jesse?"

"No! I'll put a contract out on 'em! Let 'em mess with me!"

"Contract? What contract?"

"Oh, nothing, Mrs. Hutchinson, nothing."

Now, I'm not knocking the show. It was written, directed and produced really well. But the underlying current of worldly attractions was becoming a danger to me. It was weaning me from God, holiness and heaven. I was absorbing what they were showing.

It is important to watch what you put before your eyes. The world has many attractions, but those attractions can become dangerous if we become fully absorbed in them. Instead of being purged into purity by the Spirit of God, we may end up being weaned, ever so slowly, away from the Lord.

After a while, you become conditioned to hearing cursing. You become conditioned to watching adultery on television. Things that used to bother you as a believer become more common, less threatening and easier to digest. Ever so slowly, you become conditioned to the way the world thinks. And that isn't good for your soul, which is your mind, your will and your emotions.

It is usually done through the great god of "entertainment." Remember that there is nothing wrong with having fun or being entertained. I'm all for that. But watch out what you allow yourself to digest. You can be laughing and not even notice the underlying current that is in direct opposition to what you believe. You can hear a point of view so much that it seems kind of OK. Watch that.

I'm not saying you shouldn't watch this or that. All I'm saying is to be aware and keep your heart pure. Some people really take in what they see, while others just don't. Only you and God can judge what you can see and what you can't. Only you and God can judge what you can hear and what you can't. That is between you and God. I encourage you to just step back a bit and recognize what you're taking into your heart.

Remember that most of the people in the entertainment world don't know God. They're coming from a lost and confused point of view. Many do things to deliberately shock you—to go against the grain just to grab your attention. Attention in their world means money. Understand that, and then seek to keep your own heart pure. You don't have to allow any of their impurity to find a home in your heart. Whatever you see or hear doesn't have to influence you, because the greater power is in you!

You can recognize any impurity and choose to avoid it.

Greater Is He Who Is in You

You may have a defect in your life, a stumbling block that needs purging. I know that there are some people who have a hard time going into a convenience store without lusting after the bottle of whiskey behind the counter. If you've felt that way, it's important to realize that alcohol is controlling you and you need deliverance from it. Nothing should control you but God. You're stronger than that! Greater is He who is in you than he who is in the world! (1 John 4:4.)

But before you can be set free from the bondage of any kind of compulsive behavior and successfully resist the devil, you've got to want to give up the habit. Although God can help you, He will not force Himself on you. He will only help when He is asked in faith. It's crucial that you make a clear-cut decision by asking yourself, "Do I want to keep doing this?" or "Do I really want to change? Do I want to turn from my ways and begin to follow the Lord Jesus instead?"

Don't kid yourself either. Be honest. Be sure that you are not playing games but that you are serious about making a change in your life. And don't worry. You don't have to kick anything completely on your own. Just admit to yourself that you have a problem and you need Jesus to help you with it. Really, it doesn't matter whether a person is struggling with drugs, alcohol, pornography, gambling or food. No one can give up anything successfully without the aid of Jesus! So you're no different than anybody else. We all need Jesus' help in our lives! Cut yourself some slack with the condemnation, and just open up to God about it.

Before I was saved, I was an extreme guy. I was going to hell with gusto! But when I decided to give my life to the Lord Jesus, I decided that I wasn't playing games. I needed help, and I knew it! The night when Jesus came into my life, I was cleansed of all sin, and I was totally delivered from bad fruit. Although I had to go play in a club that night, I walked on the stage a saved man. I didn't look any different. I didn't even smell different; alcohol was still on my breath. But I was different! God had changed me inside!

It is important to make a quality decision to start abiding and stick to what God says when you need deliverance. If you want to be delivered, you must want to give the problem to Jesus. You must *want* to give your life and this problem to Him.

Now, some people say that it's good to gradually taper off whatever they're addicted to, and maybe that works for them. But I don't really agree. I believe the best way to quit doing something is to quit! Make a decision, and allow Jesus to remove the root of that thing—and then stick like glue to what He's done for you!

For me, the day I was born again was the day I stopped being a womanizer, alcoholic and drug addict. That was it. But God could never have helped me unless I wanted it. I had the power to go against His change in my life. Psalm 106:43 NIV illustrates this when it says, **Many times he delivered them, but they were bent on rebellion and they wasted away in their sin.**

I could have gone out a week later and gotten falling-down drunk if I'd wanted to. I could have taken pills or snorted cocaine and wasted away in sin. I could have committed adultery. But I didn't want to! Why? Because I'd been purged! God had done too much in me for me to turn back! And because I made the decision to turn away from my old life, God honored me and took away my compulsive and obsessive behaviors concerning alcohol and drugs. He did it the minute I gave the problem and my life to Him! Although the devil came to tempt me later, because of my commitment to God I was able to resist the temptation and continue in my new life.

Can God take away all your compulsive desires and give you the strength to say no to temptation? Yes. He can do that. He did it for me. I know He will do it for you.

God Will Replace Impurities With Principles

When the Lord begins purging you of impurities, He begins replacing those former impurities with new principles. You become a person of principle concerning that area. Then when the devil comes, you're able to say no because you're a person of principle!

Once a man asked me, "Jesse, you know you're on television a lot. Now, I've been to several of your meetings, and a lot of women follow you around."

"You've noticed that?"

"Yeah, I've noticed that. Does that bother you?"

"No, that doesn't bother me."

"What makes you think you won't fall, Jesse?"

That was a good question. But, you see, I am a dead man. I'm crucified with Christ daily, not just on Sundays. The reason I've been successful in avoiding all that mess isn't that I have some great ability to say no, because I'm just as human as anyone else is. I can because the Lord delivered me from that impurity. He plucked that bad fruit right off me and replaced it with something called principle. For me, it's the principle now. When sin shows itself to me in the way of temptation, the first thing I think of is, *What would God think about that?*

Now, I'm not the ugliest man in the world. I've got white hair, and I travel a lot. Some women think that if you've got white hair, a suit and a briefcase, you must have money. And money is the biggest turn-on to a lot of people. It's true. You would be surprised how many women swoon at the thought of money. You just have to look reasonable, and they'll try to hook up with you.

You just have to go to Kennedy Airport and hang around for fifteen minutes at the baggage claim with a suit and a briefcase. If you look reasonable, some mama will come up to you and say, "What's happening? First time in New York?" Before you know it, it's all up to you to say yes or no. But I've learned some things through my relationship with God and reading His Word. I've decided that I will not allow my flesh to rule my life. Why? Principles. God has given me principles that now take precedent over the flesh.

Joseph had them too. When his boss' wife hit on him in Genesis 39, he refused to sleep with her. He told her, **How then can I do this great wickedness, and sin against God?** (v. 9). Joseph was a man of principles. That particular impurity had been purged out of his life some time before, maybe when he was in prison. But even before that, he had a chance to steal, and he refused to steal. He wanted to be a good worker. He was a man of principles.

If You Don't Embarrass Sin, Sin Will Embarrass You

I think I sort of know what Joseph felt like. I remember one time I was on a plane when a woman approached me. It was a Saturday night, and I remember that because I very seldom fly on a Saturday night.

I was sitting in an aisle seat and had just gotten a *USA Today* paper. I was reading an article and trying to figure out how much the president was going to charge me in taxes. My mind was immersed in it.

About a minute before the airline staff closed the door, a beautiful woman came flying in to get her seat. I glanced up and then back down at the paper as she started toward her seat. It was right next to mine. Suddenly she hit my knees. It kind of startled me, so I looked up at her.

She looked down at me, smiled and said, "Aren't you glad you're sitting by me?"

That shocked me. I said, "Ma'am?"

She repeated herself, "Aren't you glad you're sitting by me? I sure like your hair. Where are you going?"

I thought to myself, *That's a stupid question, woman. You're on the same plane I am. You ought to know where we're going.* Then it hit me. She was putting the make on me! I was still kind of shocked. I said, "What?"

"We could make beautiful music together," she whispered. "If you've got time, I've got time."

Now, I could see the men sitting across the aisle from me smiling at this. They were listening to every word and panting like dogs. They started going, "Oh! Oh! Oh! Oh!" I just looked at her, and I started closing my newspaper.

"If you've got time, I've got time." I heard the words again.

I smiled at her and sat silently for a moment. Then I got an idea. I decided to embarrass what was embarrassing me.

I raised my finger to point at her, and I loudly said, "Whore of Babylon! Whore of Babylon! Whore of Babylon! Whore of Babylon! Whore of Babylon!"

"Ah!" she gasped, sucked in her breath and ran to the back of the plane. I had embarrassed the socks off her!

The funniest part was these two men beside me. I heard one of them say, "Where's Babylon?" They wanted to know where Babylon was.

Now, how did I resist? That woman was blatantly trying to pick up on me. She didn't care if others heard, and she was enjoying the flirting process. How could I resist? Because I'm some great man of faith? No! I can resist because I've been purged from those impurities. According to Galations 2:20-21,

I am crucified with Christ: nevertheless I live; yet not I, but Christ liveth in me: and the life which I now live in the flesh I live by the faith of the Son of God, who loved me, and gave himself for me. I do not frustrate the grace of God: for if righteousness come by the law, then Christ is dead in vain.

This body is full of the Spirit of God, and sin does not fit! I abide in Him, and His Word abides in me. Suddenly principles arise.

The lady never came to the front again. She stayed in the back for the rest of the flight, and I didn't even see her when we landed. People have told me, "Well, I wouldn't have done it that way, Jesse." Do you know how I respond? I say, "If you don't embarrass sin, sin will embarrass you."

If temptation is getting in your face, embarrass it! Do whatever it takes to resist so that the devil can flee! Your ego means nothing. Don't let temptation stroke it. Embarrass that sin, and you won't have a problem resisting it. You'll stop it right in its tracks! I believe that if some of the preachers who have fallen had embarrassed sin, they wouldn't have fallen and lost their ministries over some crazy night of lust. It is ridiculous to let some stupid sin destroy your life.

Now, I could have said, "What's happening, Mama? Get down with your bad self," and thought to myself, *Whoa! I still got it, Jack.* But the principles within me would not allow that to happen. I've received Christ's nature.

Jesus Christ dealt with this same sort of thing. The Bible says that He was tempted in all mannerisms of men. Isn't lust for women a "mannerism of men?" Sure it is. Do you think Mary Magdalene was following Jesus just to hear Him preach? There were sex scandals in Jesus' day too. Believe me, things haven't changed that much.

Magdalene means "seashore." Mary worked the docks. The girl was in the business of selling her body. Jesus and His disciples were always getting boats and traveling. I don't recall reading a Scripture where Jesus looked at Mary and said, "What's happening, Mama? How much?"

Jesus was clean. He was a man of principles. Yes, He was tempted, but He didn't allow temptation to get very far. He always spoke directly about sin. He didn't take advantage of people. He looked at Mary and saw a lost, hurting soul—a sheep without a shepherd. He saved her, and then guess what? She began to follow Him.

Can't you hear the religious hierarchy? I can imagine their saying, "I tell you what, Reverend Jesus, I wouldn't allow that to happen. You know how that looks, that prostitute following You around. It looks like You've got something going on on the side, know what I mean?"

But Jesus didn't care about that. He gave Mary Magdalene the greatest commission of any person in the Bible. After the crucifixion it was Mary who saw Him and ran down the road declaring, "He's alive!" That was a high honor. Why did Jesus choose her to see Him first? Because He had principles. He wanted to show that even those who are cast aside by the world are considered great in His sight.

You Can Be Free From Lust

Jesus knew how to handle temptation. One temptation that seems to be the quiet sin of men and women today is lust. It's the secret problem many people deal with on a day-to-day basis.

You may be a born-again man who can't stop your eyes from bugging out of your head and lust from forming in your heart when a beautiful woman walks by. Sure, you're a man. I know she's a woman! But that doesn't mean you're supposed to turn into a panting dog, drooling all over the floor. God didn't make women just so men could lust after every good-looking one who walked through the door.

Now, I'm not saying you shouldn't notice beauty. Don't let the pendulum swing completely the other way. There is nothing wrong with recognizing beauty in all of God's creation, including women. But there is a heart issue here when lust gets involved. Women are more than just a bunch of parts. They're people whom God created. If you're lusting after women, you've got a defect, a bad piece of fruit hanging off your branch, and you need to allow God to purge you of the root of that problem.

Lust is nothing to be ashamed of. It's just something to be delivered from. And nobody has to know about it but you and God. Remember that you're stronger than any kind of lust. God can change your heart! He is a big God. He created your sexuality. So He sure can fix it up if it's going in the wrong direction. He can sure bring it back in line if it has gotten over into lust or perversion.

Jesus talked pretty straight about lust. He said that if you had lust in your heart for a woman, in His eyes you'd already slept with her. You'd already committed adultery. And that is serious business to God. If you're a woman, the same goes for you. Whoever you are, if you've got a problem with lust or perversion, God can take care of it. He can purge you of every impurity.

When Jesus took your infirmities, the Bible says that He took your iniquities too. (Isaiah 53:5.) Iniquity is just another word for rebellion. It is another way of saying that Jesus delivered you from rebellion against God and His ways. Addiction isn't God's way. Lust isn't God's way. Sickness isn't God's way. Why do you think Jesus healed people so many times and said, "Your sins are forgiven," when He did it? Because all of it—sickness, addiction, lust—is about rebellion. It's just that in sickness, your body is rebelling against God's way, and in lust, your mind is rebelling against God's way. Anything that isn't faith is sin. (Romans 14:23.) That is the bottom line.

You can let the purity of the Gospel touch you as far as the pollution of this world has. You can allow God's precious Spirit to invade those rebellious cells and command them to line up with the Word. This isn't fairy tale stuff here. It's true. It's powerful. And it's within your reach.

As a Dog Returneth to His Vomit, So a Fool Returneth to His Folly

There are some bad pieces of fruit that God purges us of that we may continually be drawn back to. If you're struggling with one, let me give you a Scripture that may help you out a bit. Proverbs 26:11 says, **As a dog returneth to his vomit, so a fool returneth to his folly.** Gross, isn't it? What is your folly? What is your stumbling block? Do you return to it?

Temptation will come. Satan will make sure of that. James 1:13-15 warns us,

> **Let no man say when he is tempted, I am tempted of God: for God cannot be tempted with evil, neither tempteth he any man: but every man is tempted, when he is drawn away of his own lust, and enticed. Then when lust hath conceived, it bringeth forth sin: and sin, when it is finished, bringeth forth death.**

Sin is vomit in the eyes of God. And it all starts with temptation. Temptation comes, but then you are the one who chooses whether you will be drawn away by your own lust. If you are, that lust will conceive. You'll be pregnant with it! And eventually you'll give birth to sin. What happens then? When sin is finished with you, then it will bring forth death in your life. It will rob you of the life of God.

That is what sin does to a person. I always like to say this: Sin will take you further than you want to go, keep you longer than you want to stay, charge you more than you want to pay! Death—that is the wage of sin. And does death sound like something you want? OK, then here is a practical bit of advice for combating temptation. The next time you start to move back toward that impurity in your life, try this: Think of Proverbs 26:11.

Imagine that impurity in your mind as a big pool of steaming vomit. Then imagine yourself going back to that pool of vile stuff to lap it up! Oh yeah, visual images like that may be disgusting. You may shudder at the thought of it, but I'll guarantee you this—you won't forget it!

And you'll be one step closer to saying no to Satan and all his works. If you picture vomit enough, you'll run from that impurity! You won't be able to get away fast enough! Hey, it works for me! It is called resisting. James put it this way: **Submit yourselves therefore to God. Resist the devil, and he will flee from you** (James 4:7).

Submitting yourself to God requires purging. Resisting the devil requires a decision to do it. Before you can get rid of something, you must want to be free of it.

Sometimes Our Acceptance of the World's Trash In Our Lives Keeps Us From Receiving God's Best

This world has many attractions. The problem is that often they become distractions from the things of God in your life. Let's just face it. In your life, how many times have you gone up to the altar for healing? Have you gotten healed every time? No, probably not. Most people don't. If you're sick now, aren't you tired of getting prayed for and not receiving the healing you need? Sure you are. I know that if I were sick and I'd been prayed for more than once, I'd consider that one time too many! Why can't we receive the first time? Why is it that sometimes healing comes and sometimes it doesn't?

I don't believe that it is always a lack of faith. I don't believe that it is always an abundance of unbelief. Sometimes, I believe that it is about purging. There may be some purging going on. Sometimes you got healed, and sometimes you stayed sick. There may have been some defects, some stumbling blocks, in your way.

Now, I'm not saying defects are enough to keep you from heaven, but they are enough to stop the flow of God's power in your life. They are enough to stop God's power to break natural law in your situation. Something hinders your healing.

The world and all its trash can distract us and fill us with things that need to be purged from our hearts so that we can receive from God. It's the trash that plugs up our hearts and contaminates our minds with confusion that often blocks the flow of God's power. And that's why the need to purge is so great.

CHAPTER 11

Doing Whatever It Takes

There are some Scriptures in the Bible that I just don't like. Look at Matthew 5:44, for instance, **Bless them that curse you—** there is a good one. **Pray for them which despitefully use you**—oh yeah, I want to do that! Those verses are like eating sauerkraut to me. I read it and get a bad taste in my mouth! I think, *Augh! Why would I want to pray for somebody who is cutting my guts out? I want to beat his brains out! I want to beat him and repent later!*

Now, maybe those Scriptures aren't too terribly hard to deal with when someone is just talking badly about you, but what if you caught your spouse in an affair? Could you pray for the other person involved? Whoa! That is when this stuff gets serious!

Would you say, "Oh, Jesus! Lord, I know that little tart stole my husband of twenty years. I know she's twenty-two and he's forty-four, Lord, but would You just save her, Lord? Save her, Lord!"

You wouldn't pray like that now, would you? You'd probably scream, "Lord! Kill her! Rip her false fingernails off her fingers! Let all her hair fall out the next time she gets her hair done. Lord, let cellulite break out like an epidemic on her body! And kill that superficial idiot husband of mine while You're at it, Lord!"

Pray for them which despitefully use you. It gets really hard in a situation like that.

When your kids curse you out or your family speaks evil of you, **bless them that curse you** gets kind of hard. It is never easy. It's natural to want to kill the woman who broke up your marriage. It's natural to want to spew words of anger back at your teenagers when they're vomiting hateful words at you; it is natural to want to rear back and slap the fire out of them when they cuss at you. It's natural to want to knock people in the head when they're spreading vicious rumors about you. It's natural! It's natural! It's natural! But do you know what the problem is with this situation? God isn't natural. And now that you're born again, you aren't natural either!

Jesus' Teaching Is All of His Words— Not Just the Ones We Like

Does that mean you can rip those verses out of the Bible just because you don't like them? No. If I want the promises in the Word, I know that I have to accept Jesus' words as His whole teaching. *All* of Jesus' words are for me. *All* of His words are for you.

If we're going to receive it *at all*, we must believe it *all!* Doing that breaks the power of natural law. You really do break the power of nature when you choose to obey God's Word in life's situations. Will you always like listening to Jesus' whole teaching? No. Should you do what He says anyway? Yes. You don't have to like it; you just have to do it. That's just one more way to break natural law in your life. That's one more way to produce good fruit on the earth.

There Are Conditions To Receiving the Promises of God

You see, there are conditions to receiving the promises of God. I call them the "ifs" and "thens" of the Bible. *If* you believe, think or do the

Word, *then* you can expect to receive what the Word has promised you. If you research healing in the Bible, you'll notice that although sometimes the subject is mentioned as direct commands from the Scriptures and others are Bible stories that illustrate some of the ways God has healed in the past, all are based on conditions—God's conditions.

Want Healing? Do Whatever It Takes!

Take Exodus 15:26, for instance. There it says,

> **If thou wilt diligently hearken to the voice of the Lord thy God, and wilt do that which is right in his sight, and wilt give ear to his commandments, and keep all his statutes, I will put none of these diseases upon thee, which I have brought upon the Egyptians: for I am the Lord that healeth thee.**

God's people needed to abide! They needed to listen to God and do what was right. He told them to listen to His commandments and to do them.

This Scripture showed that if God's people obeyed Him, then He would keep them from disease. Although we are under a new and better covenant because of Jesus' shed blood on the Cross, we still must obey God if we want to receive anything from Him. If we want healing, we still must be prepared to do what it takes to get it. *Whatever it takes!* That's my motto in this ministry, and I think it's a great motto for going after anything from God.

Unforgiveness Is a Condition, and It Will Stunt the Flow of God's Power

I'm sure you've noticed that forgiveness seems to be attached to healing a lot in the Scriptures. In Numbers 12:1-16 there is a story about Moses' sister, Miriam. Miriam had leprosy, and she could have been healed a lot earlier than she was. What delayed her healing? A bad attitude—that's what.

What did Miriam do? She spoke against God's man, Moses. Miriam and Aaron were irritated because Moses married out of his race. He married an Ethiopian, and Miriam didn't want to listen to him because of it. But Moses was God's servant. He was their leader because God had made it so.

Verses 1 and 2 show the attitude Miriam and Aaron had about the situation: **And Miriam and Aaron spake against Moses because of the Ethiopian woman whom he had married: for he had married an Ethiopian woman. And they said, Hath the Lord indeed spoken only by Moses? hath he not spoken also by us? And the Lord heard it.**

They were thinking, *Why do we have to hear from God through just Moses? Hasn't God spoken to us?* This was obviously not too pleasing to God, and Miriam kept that leprosy she contracted until she got her heart right. This shows that it's possible to hinder our own receiving by our anger and bad attitudes toward others. Miriam needed purging! This story illustrates the role repentance has to play in healing. It is possible to be saved but have anger or bitterness in your heart, which prevent your own ability to receive healing. And that is why it's so important to be purged of it!

Jesus Is the Embodiment of the Healing Rod of Moses

Numbers 21:7-9 shows how God's people were inflicted with a plague of snakes because of the words of their mouths. They murmured against God and Moses, and then the snakes came.

> Therefore the people came to Moses, and said, We have sinned, for we have spoken against the Lord, and against thee; pray unto the Lord, that he take away the serpents from us. And Moses prayed for the people. And the Lord said unto Moses, Make thee a fiery serpent, and set it upon a pole: and it shall come to pass, that every one that is bitten, when he looketh upon it, shall live. And Moses made a serpent of brass, and put it upon a pole, and it came to pass, that if a serpent had bitten any man, when he beheld the serpent of brass, he lived.

You can still see this symbol in medical facilities today. And it is thousands of years old! What it symbolizes is God's power to heal when we simply look to Him in faith. Jesus referred to Himself as the embodiment of the rod in John 3:14-15 when He said, **And as Moses lifted up the serpent in the wilderness, even so must the Son of man be lifted up: that whosoever believeth in him should not perish, but have eternal life.**

Here Jesus proved that when He would be lifted up on the Cross, whoever would believe on Him and his work at the Cross wouldn't perish but would have eternal life. By aligning Himself with the healing rod of Moses, Jesus proved that He was the new healer. For us today this means that by looking to Jesus' work at the Cross we can boldly declare that by His stripes we are healed.

Releasing Pride and Submitting Your Body to the Lord

Another "whatever it takes" example of healing is the story of Naaman and his seven dips in the disgustingly muddy and dirty Jordan River. Second Kings 5:1-15 shows how God deals with a person who is innocent or ignorant of the wrongdoing that can sometimes cause sickness.

The Bible says that Naaman's master thought Naaman was a great and honorable man because by him the Lord had given victory to Syria. He had served his country well, yet even though he was a great man, he contracted leprosy. Naaman's wife's maid was vital in his healing, because it was she who told him about seeking out the prophet Elisha. This shows us how important it is for us to tell others what we know about God and His work. They may be foreigners to God's ways, and we can be vital to their success!

For us, this story shows that sometimes God's ways are much different than ours. In this story, God unearthed pride in Naaman by telling him to do something that a man of his stature would normally never do. When he released the pride and submitted to God's way, he was supernaturally healed. Natural law broke just as Elisha had said it would! Naaman was cleansed of all pride *and* all leprosy!

Sickness Can't Stay in the Presence of God

Psalm 91:9-10 shows us another condition concerning healing. There it says that *if* we make the Lord our habitation, *then* we will have protection from sickness and contagious disease:

> **Because thou hast made the Lord, which is my refuge, even the most High, thy habitation; there shall no evil befall thee, neither shall any plague come nigh thy dwelling.**

Here is yet another Scripture proving the power of intimacy with God. If you get close enough to the Father, your body won't be able to keep sickness or disease. Sickness and disease must flee in the presence of the Most High.

Think about heaven. When you get there, there won't be any sickness or disease. Why? Because neither can exist in the presence of God. Immediately, they must flee!

"Oh, but that is heaven, Brother Jesse," you might say. Yeah, that is heaven, but did you know that we're supposed to pray and believe for God's will to be done on earth just as it is in heaven? Reread the "Our Father" prayer, and you'll see that Jesus Himself implemented this type of thinking. Matthew 6:9-10 says, **After this manner therefore pray ye: Our Father which art in heaven, hallowed be thy name. Thy kingdom come.** *Thy will be done* **in earth, as it is in heaven.**

That's something to think about, isn't it?

Jesus Took a Stroll on the Sea of Galilee

When Jesus lived on earth, He was interested in fulfilling the Father's will **in earth, as it is heaven.** He broke the power of natural law with His faith and with His will. For instance, consider the time He took a stroll on the Sea of Galilee. (Matthew 14:22-33.)

It didn't matter to Jesus that it was water, not land. It didn't matter to Him that He'd known all His life that water isn't a hard surface. Jesus strapped on His sandals and started hooking it—and in the middle of a storm, too!

Do you remember the story in Matthew about Jesus walking on the water? Let me give you a little recap if you don't. It was right after Jesus fed the 5000. Now, you'd think after seeing such a miracle that the disciples would be raring to go in faith. Nope.

After the people were fed and the service was over, Jesus told His disciples to get into the boat and go to the other side. That was His command—"Go to the other side!" He told them that He would take care of the people and send them away. Verse 25 says, **And when he had sent the multitudes away, he went up into a mountain apart to pray: and when the evening was come, he was there alone.**

Jesus had spent the rest of the day praying on the mountain, and when it got dark He decided to leave. In the meantime, a storm was brewing on the sea.

The sea was tossing the disciples' boat around, and the wind was whipping back and forth. Some of those men were fishermen and were used to being on the sea, but a storm was a storm. Nobody exactly liked it, and it was always dangerous. It was then that Jesus decided to go take a look at what was going on with His boys.

The disciples were smack-dab in the middle of the storm when they saw a man walking toward them—on the water. Panic started on the boat. The disciples were just plain scared. They'd never seen a man walking on water before. And in the middle of a storm with the wind wailing and the boat swaying, He looked like a ghost floating on top of the water!

They started screaming. The Bible says, **They cried out for fear** (v. 26). I can imagine what those boys were crying out. I can just hear them screaming, "Ahhhhhhh! It's a ghost! And it's walking *toward* us! Ahhhhhhh!"

Now, what did Jesus do when He looked across the water at those crazy, screaming disciples? He said, **Be of good cheer; it is I; be not afraid** (v. 27). In other words, "Cheer up! It's Me! Relax; there is nothing to be scared of." The Scriptures don't say that He hollered back, so He was probably getting pretty close. Obviously, He was close enough for them to hear Him, because verse 28 says that Peter responded to Him: **And Peter answered him and said, Lord, if it be thou, bid me come unto thee on the water.** Peter was testing the water, so to speak. He was giving a condition. Now, he called Jesus "Lord," but in the same breath he said, "*If* You really are who You say You are, ask me to meet You out there."

What did Jesus say? One word: **Come** (v. 29).

Peter stuck his leg out of the boat! Now, buddy, that takes faith! The Bible didn't say that Peter stuttered and shuddered and begged for more concrete evidence that it was Jesus. It says, **And when Peter was come down out of the ship, he walked on the water, to go to Jesus** (v. 29). Of course, you know the rest of the story.

> **But when he saw the wind boisterous, he was afraid; and beginning to sink, he cried, saying, Lord, save me. And immediately Jesus stretched forth his hand, and caught him, and said unto him, O thou of little faith, wherefore didst thou doubt? And when they were come into the ship, the wind ceased. Then they that were in the ship came and worshipped him, saying, Of a truth thou art the Son of God.**
>
> MATTHEW 14:30-33

When You Add *Your* Conditions to God's Conditions, You Stop His System of Faith From Working for You

Now, what would you do if you needed to check on some friends in the middle of a lake in a bad storm? You would probably try to rent a boat! But Jesus—He decided to break natural law. I recapped this story because I believe it illustrates the way Jesus broke natural law on behalf of His disciples.

"But that was Jesus, Brother Jesse," you might say. What's my answer to that? Peter!

Jesus hadn't even gone to the Cross yet for Peter. Yet Peter, at the Lord's bidding, jumped out on the sea and started to walk. Peter broke the power of natural law when the Lord bid Him *come.*

He made it for awhile, but then what happened?

Conditions—that's what happened!

Peter stepped out by faith, but then the conditions of the weather came in and stole his faith. Instead of focusing on the faith word from Jesus' lips, *Come,* Peter started looking at the waves. He started looking at the wind. The circumstances surrounding him caused him to become fearful again. What did he do? He began adding conditions. But faith can't have conditions. It must be pure to work. Natural law just won't break when faith is squashed because of the conditions of the situation. That is why Peter started to sink.

But did you notice that Jesus immediately stretched out His hand to Peter? He immediately caught him! And what were the first words He told him? **O thou of little faith, wherefore didst thou doubt?** (v. 31). Jesus was basically saying, "Peter, you had it! You were doing it! Why did you doubt? You could have kept on walking! Your faith would have held you up."

We can't put our own conditions on receiving healing. Why? Because the conditions are already set out by God in His Word. There is no negotiating when it comes to the things of God. If we add our own conditions to receiving, it won't work. Remember that connection I mentioned earlier in the book? Breaking the power of natural law in your life happens when the Word of God unites with your measure of faith. It happens when your eyes are locked on Jesus and you're walking toward Him in faith.

We All Need the Unconditional Word of God To Help Us Break the Power of Natural Law

A lot of people add their own conditions to the Word of God. They read **By [his] stripes ye were healed** (1 Peter 2:24) and try to explain it away with their own ideas. They read **As the Father hath loved me, so I have loved you: continue ye in my love** (John 15:9) and try to find reasons why they can still harbor unforgiveness toward a certain person in their lives.

They read **As the branch cannot bear fruit of itself, except it abide in the vine; no more can ye, except ye abide in me** (v. 4) and still somehow walk away thinking that they can do something on their own. They still try to do or get fruit on their own, instead of first abiding as the Scripture says.

They read **Herein is my Father glorified that ye bear much fruit; so shall ye be my disciples** (v. 8) and somehow explain away fruit bearing. They may say, "Well, I'm still a disciple of Christ! I don't have to do anything to be that! I have grace!" That is a condition of man. It has nothing to do with the Word. Yes, there is grace, but God didn't say you became a disciple by grace. It says in Ephesians 2:5 that you were saved by grace, but only a disciple or a true follower will produce fruit. (Galatians 5:22-25.)

They read **If ye abide in me, and my words abide in you, ye shall ask what ye will, and it shall be done unto you** (John 15:7) and still wonder, *How do I get my prayers answered?*

The Bible has the answers. Sometimes we don't want to accept the conditions, but God is always clear: "If you do this, then you'll get this." He isn't trying to hide anything. He wrote this book a long, long time ago.

Sometimes people ignore the Bible's conditions and make up their own. Religion is bad about this. But I don't believe that we should ever allow the religious conditions of men to change our ideas about the Word of God. Religion will try to put a cap on your receiving. Religious people explain everything away with their own experiences. Don't fall for this. Don't receive it as your own.

I've seen religious people, through their own lack of faith, try to explain to people why it is that you can't have this or that. It is as if they don't want God to look bad or something! They're trying to shield God from criticism, so they don't preach the Word for what it is.

If Isaiah prophesied Jesus' work on the Cross and God chose that to be a part of this Holy Bible, then it is true. I believe it. It works. The bank of faith awaits a draft from us.

If You Stay in the Boat of Religion, You'll Only Meet Disciples; But Get on the Water, and You'll Meet Jesus!

Jesus had a lot of faith—enough to walk on the water. Back then, He did it literally. Today, He is still doing it when it comes to His promises in the Word.

All His promises are "on the water" with Him. There is a place called "healed," "delivered" and "fruitful," and they are embodied in the anointed One, Christ Jesus. Today, you may be surrounded by frightened disciples and questioning the presence of God in your life. If so, I want to encourage you with the words of Jesus: **Be of good cheer; it is I; be not afraid** (Matthew 14:27).

You may be in a situation like Peter's. You may be saying, **Lord, if it be thou, bid me come unto thee on the water** (v. 28). "Is it Your will, Lord? Can I break this natural law, Lord? Can I come out where You are, where healing is, Lord?" Be assured that the Lord wants you to come out on the water with Him. He wants you to be healed of what is making you sick. It is His will because it is in His Word. Your healing is in Jesus, and today He is bidding *you* to come.

What Scriptures Are You Standing On?

One problem I see in the church today concerning healing is the attitude that believing for healing is passive. It's not. Peter acted on a word from Jesus. We should do the same and take Jesus *at His Word*.

I hear people tell me all the time, "Brother Jesse, I'm believing God for my healing." I say, "What Scriptures are you standing on?"

They go, "Uh, uh...." They don't know. Some of them haven't even thought about it.

There are so many Scriptures in the Bible to align your faith with. As believers, the Word of God is the foundation of our faith. If we don't know what we're standing on, we don't have faith *in* anything. If we don't believe what we're saying, don't remember what the Word says or don't do what it says to do, then we don't have real faith in God's Word. And we must have faith *in* the Word to see any kind of results.

So we must 1) know the Word, 2) believe the Word, 3) remember the Word and 4) preserve the Word by observing to do it.

My Daughter Knew, Believed, Remembered and Preserved My Word!

My daughter is grown now, but when she was a little girl, she had no problem knowing, believing, remembering and preserving my words. Jodi saw me produce for her. Consequently, she believed I always could. Then when she'd need something, she'd remind me of it. She'd keep my words alive by acting on them. Take, for instance, when we'd be in the mall.

When Jodi was small and we walked around the mall, she was always running away. The girl didn't have a lick of sense. No fear. If something interested her, she'd go. *Foom!* she was gone. We'd spend forever looking for her. We'd find her in some store playing with something.

I'll never forget one day when we went to the mall with my brother-in-law's little girl, Julie. Jodi wasn't with us for some reason.

It was just Cathy and I with little Julie. That kid walked everywhere with us. She stayed right by our side and didn't run off. I thought, *You've got to be kidding. This is great!* Julie was an obedient little girl.

Jodi was good too—it's just that she ran off all the time. She didn't care if people were looking for her. We'd find Jodi in a toy store with all kinds of stuff in her hands. She'd see us and look up like nothing was wrong and say, "Hey, can I have this, Daddy?"

It didn't matter if I said, "Jodi, I don't have any money on me right now."

She'd just look at me all confused and say, "Write a check, Dad."

Write a check, I'd think. That was my kid's answer to money problems. It didn't matter who had to work to put money in the account. All she knew was that dad was supposed to provide. Have you ever heard of El Shaddai, the God who is more than enough? Well, to Jodi, I'm El-Sha-Dad, the dad who is more than enough!

Her friends would come shopping with us, and she'd say, "Dad, we want new dresses."

"We?"

"Yeah, me and my friend."

You know I bought two dresses! I'd see a friend climbing into the car with us, and I'd think, *I'd better stop at the bank. Jodi brought a friend.*

Jodi had faith in me. 1) She knew me by my word. I told her that if she'd obey me, she'd always be happy and blessed. I told her, "Girl, if you obey me and do right by me, you'll be blessed. You'll be blessed in the city, blessed in the field, blessed going in and blessed going out! You'll be blessed in the mall and blessed in the car." I'd go on and on about it. She knew what I meant, because she heard my word!

2) She believed my word. I didn't say one thing and do another. If I told her I was going to buy something for her, she could count on it. I came through. If I told her she was going to get a spanking when we got back home, she could count on it! There is nothing like sticking to your word to make your kids respect you. If you don't follow through, your word will mean nothing. You'll get no respect.

3) She remembered my word. She didn't forget anything. If I told her something, she'd put me in remembrance of my word. "Do you remember that you said if I didn't bite my fingernails you'd give me twenty bucks?" she'd say. "Well, look at these! You can see the nails over the edge, Dad!" I'd pay up the twenty bucks.

4) She preserved my word by observing to do what I said. Now, she didn't always do what I said. But most of the time, Jodi was a good kid, and she'd obey. We only had a couple of years of hell in the early teenage years, but after that, she got her sanity back. What she did was nothing—nothing at all—compared to what I did when I was a kid. I'd leave home on a Friday night and be gone for three days straight. I was a terrible kid. Thank God, Mama's prayer—"I hope you grow up and have a kid just like you!"—didn't come to pass. Jodi messed up, believe me, but it wasn't even in the same league as what I did.

When she was little, she knew that the key to receiving from me was to *do* what I said. And I didn't ask much. I had a few rules, and if she obeyed them, everything was good. If not, she got to see my judgement side. Lying and a smart mouth didn't fly in my house. Ingratitude was a sure way of getting nothing. Obedience and thankfulness—that's what was required of her. We had some conditions!

Be a Talker, a Believer, a Rememberer and a Doer!

When you observe to do what is written in God's Word, you're obeying James 1:22: **But be ye doers of the word, and not hearers only, deceiving your own selves.** I don't care how much you know. I don't care how much you believe. I don't care how much you remember—if you don't *do* what the Bible says, you're self-deceived. What does that mean? That means that nothing is going to happen. You're speaking the Word for nothing.

I love reading about the Word and talking about the Word with other people. I think that is great. Doing these things stimulates my faith. But I don't leave my faith at the door when I go home. If I did, I'd struggle. And I struggled enough before I was saved. Now I'm in this thing to win!

I challenge you to do something about the Word that is in your heart—and keep on doing it until that promise of yours comes to pass. If you do what the Bible says, in **due season** you *will* have what it says you can have. You will reap if you faint not! (Galatians 6:9.)

Though I Walk *Through* the Valley of the Shadow of Death

Some people don't ever walk *through* the valley of the shadow of death. (Psalm 23:4.) They spend their lives *in* the valley! After all, if they're getting hit left and right and their only armor is the helmet of salvation and shield of faith, what good is that going to do? Can you beat the devil with a shield? No! The sword of the Spirit, the Word of God, is what cuts his guts out! (Ephesians 6:16,17.)

The shield of faith is your covering. Faith is what shields you from being hurt by Satan's attacks on your life, but it is the sword of the Spirit that defeats him. The Word defeats the devil. If faith seems hard, take a look at your shield. Are darts all over it? Is your faith weighed down by past attacks?

If you're tired of fighting, chances are the last attack left your shield with some darts. Take your hand and knock those things off. Let the memories of the old attacks fall to the ground. The last attack didn't take you out. You didn't perish. Let the darts fall so that your shield of faith can be light again and you can protect yourself as you walk through the valley.

Stand firm in God's strength. Stand firm in joy, and put on the whole armor so that you can **withstand in the evil day** (Ephesians 6:13). Notice, I didn't tell you to stay in the valley. I'm not going to stay in the valley! I don't tell anyone else to do it either!

I'm not stopping and building a house in the valley. I'm not going to canonize the place and build a church there. I'm going through it! As Christians, we should never let tribulation stop us from walking through the valley with God. We will walk through that problem and overcome it if we've got our armor on. If we faint not, we'll get to the other side!

Don't Faint—It Will Just Take Longer
To Get Where You Want To Go

A lot of people have a habit of fainting in the valley. They're walking along, and *plop!* they hit the dirt. They're out cold, fainting in the valley. Later they wake up, scratch their head and say, "Oh my God, what am I going to do? I'm in this terrible, dark, miserable valley! It looks like I'll never get out of here!"

Then they shake off the depression for a moment and get fired up for God. They begin quoting Scriptures, saying, "No weapon formed against me shall prosper! A thousand shall fall at my right side and ten thousand at my left, but it shall not come near me! If God be for me, who can be against me? I'm more than a conqueror!"

They begin building their faith again with the Word until *foom!* another dart flies by. They look at the dart and think, *What am I doing in this valley!* and revert to moaning, "Oh, why me?"

Suddenly, *plop!*

They've fainted again—face first in the mud.

That is just a simple illustration, but it shows you how important "keeping the faith" is. When you allow those flying darts to overwhelm you, you weaken yourself to the point of fainting. And do you realize how long it takes to get somewhere if you're fainting all along the way?

You could spend forty years in the valley with all that fainting! Galatians 6:9 warns us, **And let us not be weary in well doing: for in due season we shall reap, if we faint not.** Ephesians 3:13 reminds us, *Wherefore I desire that ye faint not* **at my tribulations**

for you, which is your glory. When you faint not at tribulations, it is your glory! That should inspire you to keep walking in faith.

You may be smack-dab in the middle of the valley of sickness, disease or addiction, but keep walking. Don't lose your joy. Don't faint. In due season you'll reap if you faint not!

What is "due season"? Well, read on to find out about all the seasons of God.

Recognizing the Four Spiritual Seasons

> To every thing there is a season, and a time to every purpose
> under the heaven.
>
> ECCLESIASTES 3:1

God created seasons. Winter, spring, summer and fall—these are the seasons that make up our year. And with each season the earth goes through change. I believe that as Christians we experience seasons in our spiritual lives as well. I've named them the winter of restoration, the buds of spring, the warmth of summer and the gathering of fall.

The Spiritual Winter—A Time of Restoration

For many, the spiritual winter is the most difficult to understand. If you've ever said something like, "I don't know what is happening. I'm praying, but I just don't seem to be getting anywhere with God lately," then you know what I mean. In my opinion, this is a time spiritually that can be compared to our season of winter.

Winter is the time of year that can feel barren and cold to many people. On the outside, most things look dead. Most trees lose their leaves. Everything gets brown and gray. It is as if most plant life just dries up and dies for the winter. But that isn't really true. It just *looks* like everything has dropped dead! Underneath the ground, however, in the deep, hidden places of the earth, life is still going strong.

You see, in winter a tree will dig its roots deeply into the earth. Why? To gain nourishment and be restored after a year's worth of producing. All year long that tree has been giving out. Leaf after leaf, flower after flower, fruit after fruit or nut after nut—whatever it was created to produce—it has been producing! You could say it has been fruitful.

When winter comes that tree says, "Whew! I've produced all I can produce! I need to fuel up for spring, so I'd better shut it down!" And as the cold winds begin to blow and the icy rain and snow begin to fall, the tree stretches its roots down deeper into the earth and begins to concentrate on the business of preservation and restoration. Leaves may fall to the ground, but sap is flowing from the roots up through the trunk and out to the branches. Life is being given at the root level.

In our lives, we go through seasons of change. And sometimes, like it or not, it's winter. Winter is a time for preservation and restoration. In this colder season, we must dig our roots deeper into God and concentrate on the business of preservation and restoration.

For a tree, the power is in the ground in which it is rooted. For us, the power is in the Word in which we are rooted.

It is through the Word that we are preserved during the harsh season of life and restored with strength and power for the next.

Don't Bail Out or Cry Out—Stick It Out!

For some people, spiritual winter is a time to either bail out or cry out.

"Bailers" see the barren situation and feel like they've been misled. They end up saying things like, "Nothing is working. This faith stuff is a bunch of junk. I'm through with believing God for this."

"Criers" see the barren situation and feel like God has forsaken them. They cry out, "Oh, God! Where are You? Why aren't You talking to me? Help me! Help me! Please!"

Neither of these is on target, because faith works and God hasn't forsaken anybody! It's just winter—a cold time in life that requires a person to stick it out and receive nourishment at the root level.

As Christians we've just got to realize that seasons change in our lives. There are times to sow and times to reap in every situation in life. There are times to give and times to be restored. There are times to enjoy the fat of the land and times to work the land for fat! Spiritual winter is one of those times—the time to exercise faith *and* patience. It is the season that lies between the fruit bearing and fruit gathering.

If you have not experienced the manifestation of God's promise in your life and you are doing everything as "right" as you know how, you may be in your spiritual winter. If so, recognize it! Then choose to stick it out by tapping into the Source so that you can receive the strengthening nourishment you need to withstand this time.

Sap begins to feed a tree at the root level. But we've got our own "sap" called the Holy Ghost! He feeds us through our spirits when on the surface nothing or no one seems to care whether we live or die. As we dig in, the Holy Spirit starts pumping rich nourishment to our roots—the area nobody sees on the outside.

If you're in winter, I encourage you not to bail out with "This stuff doesn't work!" or cry out with "Why? Why?" I encourage you to recognize where you are and begin to seek the Word for personal restoration. Make a commitment to stick it out regardless of what you see, and let patience have its perfect work. (James 1:4.) Perfect in this sense means mature. Let patience come to maturity.

Remember, a spiritual winter may not be the warmest time of the year, but it will give you the strength to produce the rest of the year. And if you're in it, there is no better time to get back to your roots than now.

Have You Got a Case of the Brown Leaf?

The winter of restoration is a very important time in breaking the power of natural law. There was a time in my own life when this season really bothered me. I am a producer by nature. I want to do something to make a difference in this world. So when my spiritual winters would come I'd struggle with restlessness. I'd feel like I'd gotten a case of the "brown leaf," and I'd say, "God, I don't feel like I'm producing anything."

You're not, He would reply.

"I'm not? Why?"

I'm restoring what you've given out all year.

Essentially God was telling me, "Don't give up! Don't give in! Relax, you're not doing anything wrong. Just keep believing in Me and My Word! I'm working on something here! I'm restoring you!"

It's good to know what's going on. It's good to know that even in the winters of life, God is still working. God is still dealing with your spirit. Knowing that I'm in winter helps me to not look at what I see. It helps me to look at what I believe. The world may say that seeing is believing, but I know the truth—believing is seeing! Soon enough seeing will come, but believing has to come first.

That's why life's dead-looking branches and brown leaves mean nothing to me. I know there is a world of life underneath the dirt.

If you're experiencing a winter season in your life that just doesn't seem to be going anywhere, get back to your roots in Jesus. Dig deeper, and allow the sap of the Holy Spirit to rise within you. The Lord will renew your strength, preserve your joy and restore your capacity to bear fruit if you stick it out and *only believe.* Soon the winds are going to change and your joy will be made full as you see the first new buds of your spiritual spring!

The Spiritual Spring—Buds of Hope and Expectation

There is nothing quite like the first buds of spring. Bare, spindly trees suddenly begin to sprout clumps of new, shiny leaves; and bright, vibrant buds of color shoot up from the ground. Clearly, spring must be one of the most refreshing times of the year.

The temperature is still a little cold sometimes, but hope is in the air because warmth is on the way! And warm weather promises one thing—new life! Production time! Beginnings of the manifestation of God's promise in your life! You could say that as the thermals change, hope and expectation come in on the first warm fronts of weather!

In the spiritual realm, this is the time that comes right after a cold season of perseverance, patience and faith in the Word of God. You've been seeking the Lord and drawing nourishment from His Word. Now hope is quickened in you, and you begin to expect that what God promised He will be faithful to perform.

You have expectation. After all, you're budding! Hope is in your heart, and your face begins to start showing it as you say, "OK, God! I'm ready to start producing again!" No longer a leafless branch, you start to display bright new leaves of expectation. It's something people around you can see. And it's attractive to them. They see you in the bud stage and just want to be around you. Meanwhile, it is just about all you can stand to wait for your flower to come into full bloom! That's what I call living on expectations and aspirations.

Wham! It's Fruit Time!

They say that there are three types of people in the earth: Those who make things happen, those who watch things happen and those who let things happen. I believe that while there is a time to watch things happen and a time to let things happen, the most important time is when you *act* on the Word of God, use your hope and tap into faith. In other words, I think it is important to act quickly when the Lord leads you to do something. Don't beat around the bush. If God tells you to do something, do it, and do it quickly!

In my services, there are times when the Lord tells me to have an altar call for certain illnesses. He may tell me to call out a name of a sickness, disease or affliction. I do it and then ask people who have that particular problem to come forward. There is such a thing as the gift of healing, and it is different than the prayer of faith. Although you need faith to receive anything from God, the gift of healing is one of the spiritual gifts mentioned in 1 Corinthians 12:9 that the Lord gives as He wills. When it is present, the anointing to heal is even stronger than usual for those who come forward in obedience.

Now, I may call out a problem that is uncommon or common. It all depends on what the Lord is leading me to say. But it never fails that after the service someone catches me and asks me to pray for that very same problem. They say, "Brother Jesse, I know you called this out, but would you pray for me now instead?"

I don't mind praying for that person; that isn't the point. I pray and believe God with the person for his healing. But the point is that when God says, "Come forward," it is important that a person heed the call. The anointing to heal is stronger when the Lord is calling on people to come forward. That is just the truth. When a group of people are standing together in faith, there is just a lot more faith! Do you understand what I mean? It is important to act when God says to act, not just when we want act. We get His best when we act on what He says to do when He says to do it.

When Jesus invited Peter to walk out on the water, Peter didn't sit back and contemplate what it meant to walk on the water. In faith he jumped out of the boat! Sometimes you've just got to stop thinking for awhile and act. I'm not talking about being stupid and jumping out of the boat when God hasn't called you. If Jesus isn't telling you to do something, don't do it! I'm simply talking about moving when God says, "Move!" and speaking when God says, "Speak!"

When you're in spiritual spring, you're full of hope and eager to do what God says. You're like Peter. You say, "Whatever You want, God! If it's You, tell me to come out on the water. I'll jump if You say jump, God!" Because of this kind of hope and expectation, you start spilling over into the realm of faith. And when your hope turns to faith, watch out! Buds start coming! Fruit starts growing in your life!

You don't just hope it will happen—you begin to watch it happen right before your eyes! *Wham!* God comes on the scene and produces fruit on your branch! It's a time of excitement and rejoicing as the manifestation of God's promise comes to pass in your life! Suddenly you're not the only one enjoying the fruit, but others are too! This is an exciting time to be in, and it ushers you directly into the next spiritual season of your life—summer!

The Spiritual Summer—Warmth Makes the Heart Full

There is nothing like the warmth of summer. After a cold winter and the bristly excitement of spring, summer comes just in time to relax you. Summer brings a feeling of contentment as you stop and just enjoy life for awhile. Spiritual summer is much the same way. It's a time of warmth and fullness of heart—a time to rest and enjoy the goodness of the Lord.

The apostle John knew what it meant to rest in the Lord. He knew what it meant to have fullness of heart. In the Bible, the Scriptures paint us a pretty clear picture of the relationship John had with Jesus. On a personal level, it was John who seemed to be the closest to

Jesus. Although Peter, James and John are the three most mentioned together, the apostle John is repeatedly called the one **whom Jesus loved.** Now, *that's* a title, don't you think?

John 20:2, John 21:7 and John 21:20 all mention John in this favorable light. In John 13:23 we read that the apostle John was so at peace in his relationship with Jesus that he didn't even sit up in his chair! At the Last Supper, the Bible says he was **leaning on Jesus' bosom** (John 21:20). Now, that's pretty close, don't you think? John was actually leaning on Jesus' chest! He had his head on the Son of God's chest! I don't know about you, but I'd call that pretty secure in your position with Christ. I call that *close!*

You don't hear Jesus saying, "Get your head off Me, John! I'm getting hot." No! Jesus allowed it. He was close to John and didn't mind John's resting in His goodness and grace.

To me, that paints the perfect picture of the warmth and contentedness of a spiritual summer. John had walked and talked with Jesus. He'd experienced what it meant to have his needs met by the Lord. He was fed physically and spiritually all through Jesus' ministering years, and by the time of the Last Supper, his heart was full of love for his Savior. He was enjoying the warmth of his personal relationship with Jesus.

Spiritual Summer Is a Time To Reflect on the Goodness of the Lord!

The season of spiritual summer is a time of enjoying your fruit! It's the time to reflect on how the Lord has used you to help others and to be thankful for what He has done in your own life. God is good, and if you don't believe it, just ask Him! He'll tell you!

Jesus set the record straight when He said that He came to give you life and to give it to you more abundantly. (John 10:10.) He set the record straight when He said that it was the devil who came to steal, kill and destroy in life. He said that so you'd know He is a good God who cares about you and wants to bring you to your spiritual summer—your time of enjoying the blessings of the Lord.

I am the good shepherd: the good shepherd giveth his life for the sheep.

JOHN 10:10,11

The Good Shepherd gave His life for you! He cared enough for you that He told you, "Hey, I'm not the thief! I'm not the killer! I'm here to give you life and to give it to you to the fullest!" That's my paraphrase, but it's as true as true can get. God loves you so much. He wants you to know that all good things come from Him! Every bit of fruit you produce in life you produce because He is good!

The goodness of the Lord is displayed every time you abide in Him and every time His words abide in you. It is displayed every time you bear much fruit and every time you continue in His love. The goodness of the Lord is displayed every single time your joy is made full by hearing His life-changing Word! It is Jesus who makes you joyful! It is He who blesses you to the point that you are contented and full in your heart!

Spiritual summer is a season that most people really love because it's after the restoration and the aspiration. It's after the soul-searching and abiding of winter and after the exercising of hope and faith in the spring. Spiritual summer is that special time to just sit back, lay your head on the chest of the master and feel the contentment of being full of much fruit.

The Spiritual Fall—A Time To Gather

I am the true vine, and my Father is the husbandman. Every branch in me that beareth not fruit he taketh away: and every branch that beareth fruit, he purgeth it, that it may bring forth more fruit. Now ye are clean through the word which I have spoken unto you.

JOHN 15:1-3

All the seasons of God have a clear reason, and fall is no exception. Fall is the time of gathering—the time to be made clean. It is the season in your life when the Lord gathers to Himself the much fruit you've produced in the spring and enjoyed in the summer.

As for me, I have to admit that I really like the spiritual summer! I like it when everything is going right and flowing well! I like being a branch that is heavily laden with much fruit! It looks good to have all that juicy stuff hanging off my limbs. I'm saying, "God, this is great! I'm so full! I'm ready for anything—hallelujah!" Then here comes God, and I feel that little tug on my branch. I say, "Hey, what are You doing, Lord?"

I'm taking your fruit.

"You're taking my fruit? No! Leave the fruit! Leave the fruit!"

As Christians, we don't always want to let go of our fruit! But God knows that if we don't let go of our past fruit we won't have room for more fruit. So He moves us out of the comfort zone of summer and plucks us clean of our fruit until we have room in our lives to produce more.

Jesus takes all those baskets of fruit, brings them to the throne of the Most High and says, "Angels! Look at what the redeemed of the Lord have done on planet earth!" Then He hands it to those ministering spirits and says, "Go forth and cover this earth with the abundance of my family! Cover it from pillar to post, that all may eat of My goodness!"

Never Forget the Words of the True Vine, Jesus Christ

There is a reason that you're here on this earth. You've got a purpose. You're a branch of the Most High God—a limb that is linked up to the true vine. And you can be assured that your Father, the husbandman, is well able to take good care of *you*. As you abide in Him and His words abide in you, you *can* move through the seasons of your life with confidence and in peace.

Remember, Jesus is the same yesterday, today and forever. (Hebrews 13:8.) The natural law that you seek to break isn't unbreakable. It shatters when confronted with fearless faith in the Word of God! Why? Because every word from God is *alive!* It holds immense power. It holds every answer. It holds the very essence of your existence in its words—*life!*

So choose life today. Put your faith in the God who is able—**able to do exceeding abundantly above all that** [you] **ask or think,**

according to the power that worketh in [you] (Ephesians 3:20). Lay aside your fears, and put your faith in the only words that will ever change anything at all—the Holy Word of God.

A Little Lagniappe—Scriptures To Help You Break the Power of Natural Law

In Southern Louisiana we have a word we use called *lagniappe* (\'lan-yap\). It is Cajun French for "something given gratuitously" or, as the locals would say, "a little something extra."

I've included some Scripture references below that I encourage you to look up for yourself. Read each one and allow the Holy Spirit to guide you to the ones that best suit *your* particular situation. It is my sincere prayer that the Lord will speak to you through His Word and bless you with wisdom, knowledge and power. Enjoy the lagniappe!

So Abraham prayed unto God: and God healed Abimelech, and his wife, and his maidservants; and they bare children.

GENESIS 20:17

And said, If thou wilt diligently hearken to the voice of the Lord thy God, and wilt do that which is right in his sight, and wilt give ear to his commandments, and keep all his statutes, I will put none of these diseases upon thee, which I have brought upon the Egyptians: for I am the Lord that healeth thee.

EXODUS 15:26

And ye shall serve the Lord your God, and he shall bless thy bread, and thy water; and I will take sickness away from the midst of thee.

EXODUS 23:25

And the Lord will take away from thee all sickness, and will put none of the evil diseases of Egypt, which thou knowest, upon thee; but will lay them upon all them that hate thee.

DEUTERONOMY 7:15

Then went he down, and dipped himself seven times in Jordan, according to the saying of the man of God: and his flesh came again like unto the flesh of a little child, and he was clean.

2 KINGS 5:14

O Lord my God, I cried unto thee, and thou hast healed me.

PSALM 30:2

The angel of the Lord encampeth round about them that fear him, and delivereth them.

PSALM 34:7

The Lord will strengthen him upon the bed of languishing: thou wilt make all his bed in his sickness. I said, Lord, be merciful unto me: heal my soul; for I have sinned against thee.

PSALM 41:3,4

Why art thou cast down, O my soul? and why art thou disquieted within me? hope thou in God: for I shall yet praise him, who is the health of my countenance, and my God.

PSALM 42:11

Because thou hast made the Lord, which is my refuge, even the most High, thy habitation; there shall no evil befall thee, neither shall any plague come nigh thy dwelling. For he shall give his angels charge over thee, to keep thee in all thy ways. They shall bear thee up in their hands, lest thou dash thy foot against a stone. Thou shalt tread upon the lion and adder: the young lion and the dragon shalt thou trample under feet. Because he hath set his love upon me, therefore will I deliver him: I will set him on high, because he hath known my name. He shall call upon me, and I will answer him: I will be with him in trouble; I will deliver him, and honour him. With long life will I satisfy him, and shew him my salvation.

PSALM 91:9-16

Bless the Lord, O my soul, and forget not all his benefits: who forgiveth all thine iniquities; who healeth all thy diseases.

PSALM 103:2,3

He sent his word, and healed them, and delivered them from their destructions.

PSALM 107:20

Be not wise in thine own eyes: fear the Lord, and depart from evil. It shall be health to thy navel, and marrow to thy bones.

PROVERBS 3:7,8

My son, attend to my words; incline thine ear unto my sayings. Let them not depart from thine eyes; keep them in the midst of thine heart. For they are life unto those that find them, and health to all their flesh.

PROVERBS 4:20-22

There is that speaketh like the piercings of a sword: but the tongue of the wise is health.

PROVERBS 12:18

A merry heart doeth good like a medicine: but a broken spirit drieth the bones.

PROVERBS 17:22

Surely he hath borne our griefs, and carried our sorrows: yet we did esteem him stricken, smitten of God, and afflicted. But he was wounded for our transgressions, he was bruised for our iniquities: the chastisement of our peace was upon him; and with his stripes we are healed.

ISAIAH 53:4,5

So shall my word be that goeth forth out of my mouth: it shall not return unto me void, but it shall accomplish that which I please, and it shall prosper in the thing whereto I sent it.

ISAIAH 55:11

Then shall thy light break forth as the morning, and thine health shall spring forth speedily: and thy right-eousness shall go before thee; the glory of the Lord shall be thy reward.

ISAIAH 58:8

Heal me, O Lord, and I shall be healed; save me, and I shall be saved: for thou art my praise.

JEREMIAH 17:14

But unto you that fear my name shall the Sun of right-eousness arise with healing in his wings; and ye shall go forth, and grow up as calves of the stall.

MALACHI 4:2

And Jesus went about all Galilee, teaching in their synagogues, and preaching the gospel of the kingdom, and healing all manner of sickness and all manner of disease among the people. And his fame went throughout all Syria: and they brought unto him all sick people that were taken with divers diseases and torments, and those which were possessed with devils, and those which were lunatick, and those that had the palsy; and he healed them.

MATTHEW 4:23,24

When the even was come, they brought unto him many that were possessed with devils: and he cast out the spirits with his word, and healed all that were sick: that it might be fulfilled which was spoken by Esaias the prophet, saying, Himself took our infirmities, and bare our sicknesses.

MATTHEW 8:16,17

Jesus answered and said unto them, Go and shew John again those things which ye do hear and see: The blind receive their sight, and the lame walk, the lepers are cleansed, and the deaf hear, the dead are raised up, and the poor have the gospel preached to them.

MATTHEW 11:4,5

But when Jesus knew it, he withdrew himself from thence: and great multitudes followed him, and he healed them all.

MATTHEW 12:15

And there came a leper to him, beseeching him, and kneeling down to him, and saying unto him, If thou wilt, thou canst make me clean. And Jesus, moved with compassion, put forth his hand, and touched him, and saith unto him, I will; be thou clean. And as soon as he had spoken, immediately the leprosy departed from him, and he was cleansed.

MARK 1:40-42

I say unto thee, Arise, and take up thy bed, and go thy way into thine house. And immediately he arose, took up the bed, and went forth before them all; insomuch that they were all amazed, and glorified God, saying, We never saw it on this fashion.

MARK 2:11,12

And he entered again into the synagogue; and there was a man there which had a withered hand. And they watched him, whether he would heal him on the sabbath day; that they might accuse him. And he saith unto the man which had the withered hand, Stand forth. And he saith unto them, Is it lawful to do good on the sabbath days, or to do evil? to save life, or to kill? But they held their peace. And when he had looked round about on them with anger, being grieved for the hardness of their hearts, he saith unto the man, Stretch forth thine hand. And he stretched it out: and his hand was restored whole as the other.

MARK 3:1-5

And he ordained twelve, that they should be with him, and that he might send them forth to preach, and to have power to heal sicknesses, and to cast out devils.

MARK 3:14,15

And they came over unto the other side of the sea, into the country of the Gadarenes. And when he was come out of the ship, immediately there met him out of the tombs a man with an unclean spirit, who had his dwelling among the tombs; and no man could bind him, no, not with chains: because that he had been often bound with fetters and chains, and the chains had been plucked asunder by him, and the fetters broken in pieces: neither could any man tame him. And always, night and day, he was in the mountains, and in the tombs, crying, and cutting himself with stones. But when he saw Jesus afar off, he ran and worshipped him, and cried with a loud voice, and said, What have I to do with thee, Jesus, thou Son of the most high God? I adjure thee by God, that thou torment me not. For he said unto him, Come out of the man, thou unclean spirit.

And he asked him, What is thy name? And he answered, saying, My name is Legion: for we are many. And he besought him much that he would not send them away out of the country.

Now there was there nigh unto the mountains a great herd of swine feeding. And all the devils besought him, saying, Send us into the swine, that we may enter into them. And forthwith Jesus gave them leave. And the unclean spirits went out, and entered into the swine: and the herd ran violently down a steep place into the sea, (they were about two thousand;) and were choked in the sea. And they that fed the swine fled, and told it in the city, and in the country. And they went out to see what it was that was done.

And they come to Jesus, and see him that was possessed with the devil, and had the legion, sitting, and clothed, and in his right mind: and they were afraid. And they that saw it told them how it befell to him that was possessed with the devil, and also concerning the swine. And they began to pray him to depart out of their coasts. And when he was come into the ship, he that had been possessed with the devil prayed him that he might be with him. Howbeit Jesus suffered him not, but saith unto him, Go home to thy friends, and tell them how great things the Lord hath done for thee, and hath had compassion on thee. And he departed, and began to publish in Decapolis how great things Jesus had done for him: and all men did marvel.

MARK 5:1-20

And when Jesus was passed over again by ship unto the other side, much people gathered unto him: and he was nigh unto the sea. And, behold, there cometh one of the rulers of the synagogue, Jairus by name; and when he saw him, he fell at his feet, and besought him greatly, saying, My little daughter lieth at the point of death: I pray thee come and lay thy hands on her, that she may be healed; and she shall live. And Jesus went with him; and much people followed him, and thronged him.

And a certain woman, which had an issue of blood twelve years, and had suffered many things of many physicians, and had spent all that she had, and was nothing bettered, but rather grew worse, when she had heard of Jesus, came in the press behind, and touched his garment. For she said, If I may touch but his clothes, I shall be whole. And straightway the fountain of her blood was dried up; and she felt in her body that she was healed of that plague.

And Jesus, immediately knowing in himself that virtue had gone out of him, turned him about in the press, and said, Who touched my clothes? And his disciples said unto him, Thou seest the multitude thronging thee, and sayest thou, Who touched me? And he looked round about to see her that had done this thing. But the woman fearing and trembling, knowing what was done in her, came and fell down before him, and told him all the truth. And he said unto her, Daughter, thy faith hath made thee whole; go in peace, and be whole of thy plague.

While he yet spake, there came from the ruler of the synagogue's house certain which said, Thy daughter is dead: why troublest thou the Master any further? As soon as Jesus heard the word spoken, he saith unto the ruler of the synagogue, Be not afraid, only believe. And he suffered no man to follow him, save Peter, and James, and John the brother of James. And he cometh to the house of the ruler of the synagogue, and seeth the tumult, and them that wept and wailed greatly. And when he was come in, he saith unto them, Why make ye this ado and weep? The damsel is not dead, but sleepeth. And they laughed him to scorn.

But when he had put them all out, he taketh the father and the mother of the damsel, and them that were with him, and entereth in where the damsel was lying. And he took the damsel by the hand and said unto her, Talitha cumi; which is, being interpreted, Damsel, I say unto thee, arise. And straightway the damsel arose, and walked; for she was of the age of twelve years. And they were astonished with a great astonishment. And he charged them straitly that no man should know it; and commanded that something should be given her to eat.

MARK 5:21-43

And they cast out many devils, and anointed with oil many that were sick, and healed them.

MARK 6:13

And he said unto them, Go ye into all the world, and preach the gospel to every creature. He that believeth and is baptized shall be saved; but he that believeth not shall be damned. And these signs shall follow them that believe; In my name shall they cast out devils; they shall speak with new tongues; they shall take up serpents; and if they drink any deadly thing, it shall not hurt them; they shall lay hands on the sick, and they shall recover.

MARK 16:15-18

The Spirit of the Lord is upon me, because he hath anointed me to preach the gospel to the poor; he hath sent me to heal the brokenhearted, to preach deliverance to the captives, and recovering of sight to the blind, to set at liberty them that are bruised.

LUKE 4:18

And he arose out of the synagogue, and entered into Simon's house. And Simon's wife's mother was taken with a great fever; and they besought him for her. And he stood over her, and rebuked the fever; and it left her: and immediately she arose and ministered unto them. Now when the sun was setting, all they that had any sick with divers diseases brought them unto him; and he laid his hands on every one of them, and healed them.

LUKE 4:38-40

And heal the sick that are therein, and say unto them, The kingdom of God is come nigh unto you.

LUKE 10:9

Behold, I give unto you power to tread on serpents and scorpions, and over all the power of the enemy: and nothing shall by any means hurt you.

LUKE 10:19

And when Jesus saw her, he called her to him, and said unto her, Woman, thou art loosed from thine infirmity.

LUKE 13:12

And they held their peace. And he took him, and healed him, and let him go.

LUKE 14:4

And when he saw them, he said unto them, Go shew yourselves unto the priests. And it came to pass, that, as they went, they were cleansed. And one of them, when he saw that he was healed, turned back, and with a loud voice glorified God.

LUKE 17:14,15

And whatsoever ye shall ask in my name, that will I do, that the Father may be glorified in the Son. If ye shall ask any thing in my name, I will do it.

JOHN 14:13,14

Now Peter and John went up together into the temple at the hour of prayer, being the ninth hour. And a certain man lame from his mother's womb was carried, whom they laid daily at the gate of the temple which is called Beautiful, to ask alms of them that entered into the temple; who seeing Peter and John about to go into the temple asked an alms. And Peter, fastening his eyes upon him with John, said, Look on us. And he gave heed unto them, expecting to receive something of them. Then Peter said, Silver and gold have I none; but such as I have give I thee: In the name of Jesus Christ of Nazareth rise up and walk.

And he took him by the right hand, and lifted him up: and immediately his feet and ankle bones received strength. And he leaping up stood, and walked, and entered with them into the temple, walking, and leaping, and praising God. And all the people saw him walking and praising God: and they knew that it was he which sat for alms at the Beautiful gate of the temple: and they were filled with wonder and amazement at that which had happened unto him.

ACTS 3:1-10

How God anointed Jesus of Nazareth with the Holy Ghost and with power: who went about doing good, and healing all that were oppressed of the devil; for God was with him.

ACTS 10:38

For the law of the Spirit of life in Christ Jesus hath made me free from the law of sin and death.

ROMANS 8:2

But if the Spirit of him that raised up Jesus from the dead dwell in you, he that raised up Christ from the dead shall also quicken your mortal bodies by his Spirit that dwelleth in you.

ROMANS 8:11

For the weapons of our warfare are not carnal, but mighty through God to the pulling down of strong holds.

2 CORINTHIANS 10:4

Christ hath redeemed us from the curse of the law, being made a curse for us: for it is written, Cursed is every one that hangeth on a tree.

GALATIANS 3:13

Above all, taking the shield of faith, wherewith ye shall be able to quench all the fiery darts of the wicked.

EPHESIANS 6:16

For God hath not given us the spirit of fear; but of power, and of love, and of a sound mind.

2 Timothy 1:7

For the word of God is quick, and powerful, and sharper than any twoedged sword, piercing even to the dividing asunder of soul and spirit, and of the joints and marrow, and is a discerner of the thoughts and intents of the heart. Neither is there any creature that is not manifest in his sight: but all things are naked and opened unto the eyes of him with whom we have to do. Seeing then that we have a great high priest, that is passed into the heavens, Jesus the Son of God, let us hold fast our profession. For we have not an high priest which cannot be touched with the feeling of our infirmities; but was in all points tempted like as we are, yet without sin. Let us therefore come boldly unto the throne of grace, that we may obtain mercy, and find grace to help in time of need.

Hebrew 4:12-16

Submit yourselves therefore to God. Resist the devil, and he will flee from you.

James 4:7

Is any sick among you? let him call for the elders of the church; and let them pray over him, anointing him with oil in the name of the Lord.

James 5:14

Who his own self bare our sins in his own body on the tree, that we, being dead to sins, should live unto righteousness: by whose stripes ye were healed.

1 Peter 2:24

Prayer of Salvation—Do You Know Jesus?

Or do you just know *about* Jesus? Is God a part of your life? Is He your friend? Can you talk to Him? If you've answered no to any of these questions, then I'd like to take the opportunity to introduce you to the best friend you'll ever have—Jesus!

Jesus isn't a fairy tale. He is real. He is personal. And He's ready to come into your life and help you make a change if you want Him to.

If you've never asked Him to come into your life or if you are simply not living how you should be, would you pray this prayer with me?

"Lord Jesus, I ask You to forgive me of all my sins. I confess that I am a sinner before You this day. I denounce Satan and all his works. I ask You to come into my heart and change me. Right now, Lord, I want You to know that I believe with all my heart that You are the Son of God, that You died on the cross for the sins of the world and that You rose from the dead. I confess these things with my mouth, so all of heaven and earth can hear it. I'm saved!

"Jesus, reveal Yourself to me. Reveal Your nature to me. I want to experience Your love and be whole in my spirit and my body. From this day forward I promise to include You in my life. I will tell others about You. I will walk in faith. I will excel in all that I put my hand to because I will be doing Your will, Jesus. You will be my guide and my best friend. Today I begin again. I am a new creature in You, Christ Jesus! Everywhere I go, I will let Your light shine through me.

"I pray this prayer to the Father, in the name of Jesus. Amen!"

You've just been born again! (John 3:3, Romans 10:9,10.) Shout! You made it! Your name is now written in the Lamb's Book of Life. Heaven will be your home when you die, and adventures await you from this moment on! Would you do me a favor? Write me and tell me if you prayed this prayer. Let me know that you've made Jesus your Lord!

I may never get to meet you face to face in this life. But in heaven, who knows? I might live right next door to you! If I do, I'll be at your house every day! I'll slide over on the gold streets in my socks and stick my head through your window! We'll have a great time. Until then, may the God who *breaks the power of natural law* bless you in everything you set your hand to do!

—*Jesse Duplantis*

About the Author

Jesse **Duplantis** is what some would call a true evangelist. Supernaturally saved and delivered from a life of addiction in 1974 and called by God to the office of the evangelist in 1978, he founded Jesse Duplantis Ministries with one mission in his mind and one vision in his heart—global evangelism, whatever the cost. And throughout his many years of evangelistic ministry, he has sought to do just that.

With a television ministry that spans the globe, ministry offices in America, the United Kingdom and Australia and a preaching itinerary that has taken him to over 1000 different churches to date, Jesse is still fulfilling his original call to evangelism with gusto! His commitment to Christ, long-standing integrity in ministry and infectious, joyful nature have made him one of the most loved and respected ministers of the gospel today. Oral Roberts Ministries recognized his achievements in the field of evangelism by awarding him an honorary doctorate of divinity in 1999.

A Cajun from Southern Louisiana, Jesse makes the Bible easy to understand by preaching its truths in our everyday vernacular and spicing his messages with humor. Often called the "Apostle of Joy" because of his hilarious illustrations, Jesse's anointed preaching and down-to-earth style have helped to open the door for countless numbers of people to receive Jesus as their Lord and Savior. Jesse has proved through his own life that no matter who you are or where you come from, God can change your heart, develop your character through His Word and help you find and complete your divine destiny.

To contact Jesse Duplantis

write or call:

Jesse Duplantis

P. O. Box 20149

New Orleans, Louisiana 70141

(504) 764-2000

www.jdm.org

Please include your prayer requests

and comments when you write.

Other Books by Jesse Duplantis

Heaven—Close Encounters of the God Kind

God Is Not Enough, He's Too Much!

The Ministry of Cheerfulness

Running Toward Your Giant

Don't Be Affected by the World's Message

Keep Your Foot on the Devil's Neck

Leave it in the Hands of a Specialist

One More Night With the Frogs

Running Toward Your Giant

The Battle of Life

The Return of Jesus

Available from your local bookstore.

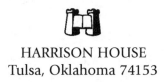

HARRISON HOUSE
Tulsa, Oklahoma 74153

The Harrison House Vision

Proclaiming the truth and the power

Of the Gospel of Jesus Christ

With excellence;

Challenging Christians to

Live victoriously,

Grow spiritually,

Know God intimately.